CORE STABILITY

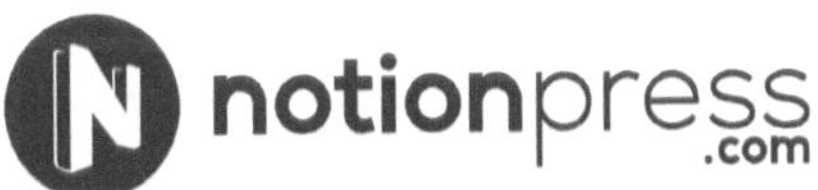

CORE STABILITY

DR.'S FITNESS-CORE STABILITY

SUKHJIVAN SINGH & HARDEEP KAUR SAINI

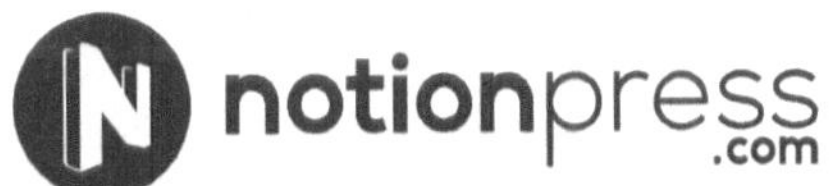

Notion Press

Old No. 38, New No. 6
McNichols Road, Chetpet
Chennai - 600 031

First Published by Notion Press 2017
Copyright © Sukhjivan Singh & Hardeep Kaur Saini 2017
All Rights Reserved.

ISBN 978-1-948230-73-5

CONTENTS

1. Core 1
2. Anatomy 4
3. Functional Core 8
4. Need 11
5. Principles of Exercising the Core 15
6. Posture 21
7. Test and Evaluation 29
8. Young Athletes 51
9. Older Adults 63
10. Bodybuilding 68
11. Weightlifting 76
12. Power Lifting 78
13. Boot Camp 81
14. Yoga 85
15. Aerobics 96
16. Mat Pilates 100
17. Strength 106
18. TRX 116

CORE

If you were to think of your body as two halves of a whole, then most likely you'd pick your waist as the midway point. This also happens to be an effective way to describe your body's core.

The body's core muscles, also known as the trunk, are made up of the transverses abdomens, lumbar multifidus, diaphragm, and pelvic floor muscles. These muscle groups encircle and support your spine making them the most intimately involved groups in spinal stabilization. They also play a crucial role in communication with the central nervous system and brain.

– According to Michelle Schwahn

In a healthy spine there is activation of deep core muscles in stabilization of the trunk before the body moves. This interaction between the deep core muscles and the nervous system plays a role in the proprioceptive feedback sent to the brain as we perform activities and undergo our normal activities.

Important

Cynthia Trentman writes in her article about Core Stability, the strengthening of functional muscle groupsleads to a more sophisticated neuromuscular system and improved lumbar spine support. Think of them as a brace for your spine. What's more, the strengthening of these muscles can lead to the reduction of urinary stress incontinence. The correlation between the transversus and pelvic floor muscles is becoming more evident.

"Many patients who have been given exercises for the transversus abdominis report a reduction in urinary stress incontinence; patients given pelvic floor strengthening exercises report a decrease in back pain."

Though they have primarily been confined to the offices of physical therapists around the globe, core strengthening exercises are slowly creeping into the depths of athletic training rooms because of their ability to refine even the most highly trained athlete. In today's aging society back pain issues are more prevalent than ever.

"In fact, eighty percent of the population experiences back pain at some point in their lives"

– Lori Evans and Tatum Wilson

In their article, At the Core, They go on to say:

"The lumbar multifidus provides segmental stabilization to the spine, which is imperative in patients with lumbar spine instability. Research shows that people with previous episodes of low back pain have delayed activation of the transversus abdominis and lumbar multifidus."

A training regimen designed to target these muscles can significantly reduce present and future pain, as well as posture problems. In addition to pain reduction and injury prevention, core stabilitycan significantly improve athletic performance. This type of training can help to teach the athletes to move more efficiently by effectively increasing the transfer of energy from core to limb.

Rick Jemmett explains this theory in his book, the Athletes Ball, to understand the concept of energy transfer, imagine a baseball pitcher who is for some reason prevented from using his lower body throughout the pitching motion; he has to keep his legs still and throw the ball using only his arm. Will he throw as hard as when he is able to use his lower body as he winds up pitching in beginning the throwing motion with the legs, kinetic energy generated in the lower half of the body is transferred through the core muscles to his throwing arm, and eventually to the ball. If the athlete's core muscles are well trained, this transfer of kinetic energy takes place efficiently. From rehab to sports and fitness training, the importance of core stability is no secret. A strong core leads to the improvement of everyday life, injury prevention, reduction, and enhanced sports performance. Growing popularity and proven results have vaulted core strengthening exercises into all types of training programs from the gym to the Pilates studio.

ANATOMY

When someone says "abs," the first thing that comes to mind for many people is the six-pack. For many, including fitness clients, the abdomen has been marginalized to include just one muscle the rectus abdominis. However, the abdominal region is composed of several key muscles that contribute to core function. The abdomen is the region lying between the proximal chest and the distal pelvis. This region is served by several muscles that contribute to spine stability in a variety of postures, providing the ability to flex, side bend, and rotate the trunk. These muscles also serve to protect the abdominal organs. Four muscles provide shape and movement to the anterior abdominal wall. Three of these muscles are described as flat muscles (the oblique and the transversus abdominis), and one is described as being strap like (the rectus abdominis).

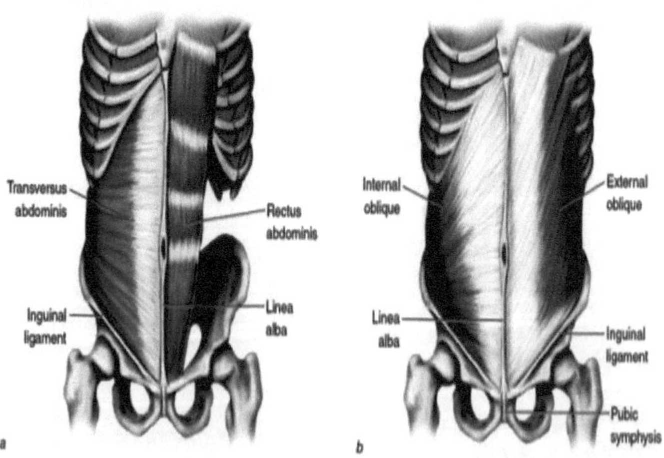

Rectus Abdominis

The rectus abdominis (RA) the muscle made famous in movies and television provides both core stability and trunk mobility. The RA is a trunk flexor. This muscle arises from the xiphoid process and adjacent costal cartilages, and it attaches distally into the pubic bone at the crest and symphysis. The RA muscle is trained when an individual performs an exercise such as the crunch.

Transversus Abdominis

The transversus abdominis (TA) is the deepest of the three flat abdominal muscles. The TA originates from the lower six costal cartilages, the thoracolumbar fascia, and the iliac crest; this muscle attaches medially at the linea alba. The TA is reported to play a significant role in core stabilization, especially during rehabilitation.

Obliques

The external and internal oblique muscles rotate and sides bend the trunk. These muscles also contribute to spinal stability. The external oblique is the most superficial muscle of the three flat abdominal muscles (the external oblique, internal oblique, and transversus abdominis). The external oblique arises from the front lateral portion of the lower seven ribs, and it inserts into the linea alba, the pubic tubercle, and the anterior portion of the iliac crest. Acting alone, the external oblique can flex the trunk, side bend the torso toward the same side (i.e., the side of the contracting muscle), and rotate the trunk toward the opposite side.

The internal oblique originates from the thoracolumbar fascia, the inguinal ligament, and the anterior iliac crest. The internal oblique also functions to provide spine stability, and it flexes and rotates the trunk toward the same side.

Muscles of the Abdominal Wall and Their Functional Actions on the Core

Sr. No.	Muscles	Origin	Insertions	Functional actions
1	Rectus abdominis	Xiphoid process and adjacent costal cartilages	Pubic bone at the crest and symphysis	Flexes and rotates the trunk
2	Transversus abdominis	Thoracolumbar fascia, inguinal ligament, iliac crest and ribs 6–12	Linea alba and public crest	Provides core stabilization, compresses abdominal wall
3	External oblique	Anterolateral (front and lateral) portion of the lower 7 ribs	Linea alba, pubic tubercle, and anterior portion of the iliac crest	Flexes the trunk, side bends the torso toward the same side rotates the trunk toward the same side
4	Internal oblique	Thoracolumbar fascia,inguinal ligament and anterior iliac crest	Linea alba and lower 4 ribs	Provides spinalstability, flexes and rotates the trunk toward the opposite side

FUNCTIONAL CORE

In anatomical terms, core stability describes the "muscular control required around the Lumbopelvic rhythm hip region to maintain functional stability." In practice, the core serves as:

1. A muscle corset that works as a unit to stabilize the body and spine with and without the movement of the limbs.

2. The centre of the kinetic chain, where the large muscle groups meet and cross into each other, providing stability for the rotating force.

3. The powerhouse, where all movements are generated from and transformed to the extremities. The main muscles involved in core stabilization can be divided into two categories:

Globalmuscles are the large muscle groups lying close to the surface. They link the pelvis to the rib cage and apart from providing general trunk stabilization, their main function is movement. These are:

External Oblique: lying on the side and front of the abdomen around the waist, helping to twist the torso.

Internal Oblique: the muscles lying beneath the external oblique, running in the opposite direction, also acting in the twisting motion.

Rectus Abdomens: is a long muscle that extends along the abdomen, in the middle section of the torso, helping to curl the trunk.

Erector Spine: is a group of three muscles running along the spine and the ribcage, from the lower back to the neck, acting when the back is in extension.

Local (postural, tonic) muscles are smaller muscle groups lying deep in the abdomen. They attach directly to the lumbar vertebrae and are responsible for providing segmental stability by controlling the lumbar segments during movement. These are:

Transverse Abdomens: the deepest lying muscle around the abdomen which acts like a corset, protecting the organs and stabilizing the spine.

Multifidus: small muscles which lie along the spine with short fibres, connecting one vertebra to the other.

Iliopsoas: two muscle groups, originating from inside the pelvis and from the

Vertebrae column join, and together exert on the femur, taking an important part in hip flexion.

Quadratus Lumborum: strings of muscles connecting the pelvic crest to the ribs and to the vertebras in the lower back, helping the side movements of the trunk.

Pelvic floor muscles: short and strong muscles lying deep at the bottom of the pelvis, responsible for letting go or holding urine. While previously the major emphasis of exercising the core has been put on strengthening the global muscles, now the theory is that both the global and the local muscle groups must be working together efficiently. Also, working on the activation and endurance of the muscle is just as important as strength, when exercising the core.

While it may be good motivation, rocking a beach-worthy body is not the only reason to get your upper body in shape. After all, your core is about more than just your abs muscles it's your body's thrust. Not only does it make easy movement, but it also houses your internal organs and central nervous system. In other words, it helps you do just about all. Here are five reasons to keep it strong.

NEED

Avert injuries

To build a strong core, it takes more than a few crunches. For Martha Purdy, a physiotherapist and Pilates instructor with Halifax Health Centre, developing a strong torso means building both core stability and core strength. "It's key to build core stability first, and then build core strength," Purdy explains. "You want to get the deeper muscles working first." Purdy says that when you've got a strong core, "everything else will fit into place on top of it," it means that your overall fitness will get better, making you less prone to injury down the road. Even though it's easy to presume that when we are moving, our extremity do most of the work, the opposite is true, most of the movements start at the centre and moves outer. A rock-solid centre will help ensure that your actions are strong and pain free. A simple but effective exercise for building core stability is to draw in the abdominal muscles, hold for five breaths, and then relax.

Protect Your Inner Organs and Central Nervous System

Staying healthy also means shielding those vital systems below the surface. Your core is not only where your organs and central nervous system do their busy work, it is also where your body's largest veins and arteries are based. Keeping strong core muscles will help ensure the whole thing stays protected as you move through your day. Renee Whitney, a

Kingston based personal trainer and owner of Focus Personal Fitness, uses the spinal cord as an example. "Your spinal cord is everything," she explains, "but if you have pressure on it because it isn't well supported by your core muscles, then it is going to affect your movements. It will eventually cause pain, and that will affect the quality of your life."

Back pain

Back pain is a general side effect of a weak core. When our abdominals are weak, it is often because our back muscles are very fragile.

Whitney

Building core strength will help bring balance to the front and back of your body. Sitting at a desk all day doesn't help, also. "Not being mindful of how sitting, and not engage our core were, can lead to things like compressed discs in our spinal cord.

Many people make the mistake of sitting for long periods with a tilted pelvis and an arched back, rather than sitting tall on their "sit bones" (think about the boney part of your bum pointing straight down). To work your core at the office, Whitney suggests sitting on a stability ball rather than a traditional chair, because the sense of instability and the movement it creates forces your abdomen to stay engaged.

Whitney

Get a Strong and Confident Posture

If your core is strong, you will be hard pressed not to carry yourself with confidence. "A tall, upright posture exudes strength,"

Whitney

"It gives the impression that this person is in control of their life." A slumped posture, on the other hand, looks weak and defeated. He suggests practicing good posture when you're in the car, by sitting up properly, and then adjusting the rear-view mirror accordingly. As soon as you start slumping, you will lose sight of yourself and you will have to sit up tall again.Once you have developed your core stability, you can start working on the more external core muscles to build strength you will be able to see. Exercises like the plank, bridge and other abdominal moves are great ways to get started. About building core strength:

"Just because you're strong, it doesn't mean you have a strong core. It's really something everyone can work on."

Purdy

The Benefits of Core Training

Tightens the abdominal structures involved in movement and improves the shift of power to and from the extremities.

Teach the muscles to work together efficiently and effectively.

The prevention of injury.

Strengthens and improves the torso's stabilization.

Improve respiratory function.

Facilitates proper division of weight and assists the body in absorption of force and transfer of forces.

Enhances neuromuscular efficiency throughout the body and neuromuscular control for efficient movement and physical position.

Improves spinal and postural organize while the body is still and in motion.

Helps to stabilize and align the spine, ribs and pelvis of a person to withstand static and dynamic force. Tightens and flattens the tummy.

PRINCIPLES OF EXERCISING THE CORE

The principles of exercising the core is a selected summary, based on what the pioneers of conditioning such as yoga, Pilates and weight training experts laid down in the past. In fact, these points can be taken as an organized statement of what is required to perform many exercise programmed effectively.

Concentration

Exercise, which does not involve the brain, is wasted. The mind must be alert at all times; controlling every movement instead of letting the body functions on automatic. Concentration is what connects mind and body and this is very important from the point of view of developing proprioceptive sense thus, injury prevention. Proprioception is the awareness of movements derived from the muscular, tendon andarticular sources, a feedback on the status of the body, the ability to adjust, compensate unexpected movements. In order to reach the optimum level of concentration, you have to be as relaxed as possible when performing your routine.

Control

In order to maximize the effect of muscle work, it is important to do the exercise exactly as described no more and no less. Apart from ensuring to focus on the particular muscle group, control is also vital in order to avoid injury. Even the simplest routine it is important to execute smooth and relaxed sets of movements with full control. Visualizing the relevant muscles working during the movement may be of great assistance for developing proper control.

Centre

When the body is functioning correctly in terms of its muscular activity the source of all the power and movement is located at the centre of the body. Energy and control for all the exercises begins in the core and flows out to the extremities. Therefore, when exercising, the primary focus should be set on the core, keeping the centre active and strong. The key to core stabilization is learning to use the deep muscles of the trunk. Activating the core means to tighten up the pelvic floor muscles, just like stopping the flow when urinating and bracing the abdomen by pulling the navel towards the spine.

Posture

Ideal postural alignment is essential for optimal human movement and performance. The spine should be in the neutral position when exercising the core. Neutral spine describes the posture that maintains three normal curves in the spine: in the neck, in the upper back and in the lower back. These three curves help to absorb stress and impact on the body while standing or sitting as well as when moving.

Breathing

In everyday life, we have a tendency to use the chest to control our breathing, using the muscles between our ribs to lift the ribcage. This is very inefficient since it does not supply new air to the lower lungs and something less than one third of the lung's surface will have new oxygen to distribute. However, with lateral breathing the lung expands outwards, thus its capacity can be increased significantly. Lateral breathing means using the diaphragm and the abdominal muscles. It is very important to coordinate breathing with the exercise, in order to establish the rhythm. The general principle is that as you prepare for the movement, you breathe in and as you perform it, you breathe out.

Timing

Repetitions of the individual exercises and the sequence of exercises should be performed as a whole unit, with continuous, flowing movements. There should be no variation of speed between exercises and the range of movement in each should be the same. While exercising, the Inhale/Exhale ratio indicates the speed and length of the movements desired (e.g.: 2:3 means that it should take approximately 2 seconds to raise, followed by 3 seconds to lower your legs).

Precision

Perfect technical execution is not an additional extra, but central to the effectiveness of the whole process. It requires a lot of time, patience and concentration. However, time and effort spent in attaining precision at the beginning will be repaid in terms of benefit. Without this precision, the value of the routine is compromised, while with practice and patience precision becomes a beneficial habit. It requires developing the ability to visualize exactly how you are moving during the exercise. Therefore, a large mirror while practicing can be very useful.

Exercise Selection

Since it requires minimum experience in training, very little space and just a few items of equipment, core stabilization exercises can be easily organized and carried out. Amongst the numberless exercises suitable to improve core stability, one has specifically selected and designed a few basic movements, which can provide an effective start when training handball players. The concept is to train the whole ranges of core muscles with exercises in different positions on the back, on the stomach and on the side. Each exercise starts with using only the body and progresses through stages with simple equipment and resistance, in order to challenge the athlete further. It is advised to master the movement of the given stage and then move on to the next level only when the existing exercise is carried out perfectly with ease and no longer challenges the body and mind.

Stages of Exercising the Core

Stage I: Core Control

Aim: To establish the training routine, learn the movements and activate the right muscles in a supported position. The most important objective of this stage is to achieve core activation and control. For building up confidence and for better control, it is advised to start the training with static exercises in a supported position, on the floor. At first, take the correct starting position with the appropriate joint alignment and neutral spine, then by pulling the navel into the spine and bracing the abdominals, activate the core. Then go through the whole range of movement with the right breathing technique and hold the position for approximately twenty five seconds before returning to the starting position. Repeat the exercise 3–4 times with twenty five second intervals. When you become confident and fluent with the technique, move from static training to dynamic repetitions, still maintaining the supported position. Go through the range of movement then return to the starting position in a 2 sec./2 sec. ratio 10 times, without break. Repeat the exercise 3–4 times with 30-second intervals.

Stage II: Core Stabilization

Aim: To maintain the training routine, to master the movements and to stabilize muscles in an unsupported position. This is the stage where proprioceptive training comes to the core. By forcing the body and mind to adjust and compensate to the unstable position, fine proprioceptive sense will develop. For building up confidence again and for better control in the changed, unsupported position it is advised to start the training with static exercises again. Adjust your body position to the equipment, maintain the appropriate joint alignment and activate your core. Go through the whole range of movement with the right breathing technique, and then hold the position for approximately 20 seconds, before returning to the starting position. Repeat the exercise 3–4 times with 20-second intervals. When you become confident and fluent with the technique, once again move from static training to dynamic repetitions, while you are in an unsupported position. Go through the range of movement then return to the starting position in a 2 sec./2 sec. ratio 10 times without break. Repeat the exercise 3–4 times with 30-second intervals.

Stage III: Core Strengthening

Aim: To modify the training routine, to master the new movements and to strengthen muscles in an unsupported position, with resistance. This is the stage to strengthen further the controlled and stabilized core. When introducing resistance training while your body is in an unsupported position, it isadvised to start with static exercises again. Adjust your body position to the equipment or resistance, maintain the appropriate joint alignment and activate your core. Go through the whole range of movement with the right breathing technique; hold the position forapproximately ten to fifteen seconds, before returning to the starting position. Repeat the exercise two to four times with ten second intervals. When you become confident and fluent with the technique, once again move from static training to dynamic repetitions, still maintaining the unsupported position. Go through the range of movement then return to the starting position in a two sec. or two sec. ratio fifteen times, without break. Repeat the exercise two- four times with thirty second intervals.

POSTURE

Good Posture

"Good posture is one in which the body is so balanced as to produce least fatigue."

– According to Avery

It means that good posture is that position of the body in which the body weight should be equally distributed over both the legs and feet as to produce least fatigue and which enables the body to function effectively. It is the balancing of body in accurate and proper manner while sitting, standing, reading, and writing or doing any other action of body

Need of Good Posture

To maintain the proper alignment of body with force of gravity as to avoid any adverse effect on the skeletal muscle structure, the human body wages a constant battle against the force of gravity. Even while we are sleeping, we change our positions a number of times to avoid discomfort. This discomfort is largely caused by pressure on the soft tissues between the bony structures and the supporting surface upon which the body is resting. Although it is possible to keep the body in such a position as to negate the force of gravity for the time being. Yet we cannot remain free from this force for a longer period. Man counteracts the force of gravity. Throughout his waking hours, much of his energy is consumed solely in the maintenance of his antigravity dynamic postures. The downward pull of gravity is a force capable of causing changes of various parts of the body when the biped position is assumed. These changes affect the skeletal system, because they change the alignment of the bony levers at various joints. Consequently, these changes cause many changes within the muscular system.

Correct posture

"There is no definite form, shape or standard for any part of the body or for the body as a whole. It is impossible, therefore, to have a definite standard as regards posture."

– Morrison and Chenoweth

"That single rigid body mechanics specification for all, regardless of body type and other factors which influence the human form, are scientifically unsupportable."

– Daniels

For each person the best posture is that in which the body segments are balanced in the position of least strain and maximum support, but even then there are, some general norms regarding postural position. These are stated below:

Standing posture

Both the heels of the feet should meet each other. Toes of the feet should be 3 inch to 4 inch apart. The whole body should be erect, straight knees, chin inside, chest forward, belly backward and pressed inside with equal body weight on both feet. For the application of the principles of stability to a standing position that is balanced and free from muscular and ligamentous strain, the line of gravity of the centre of the head, chest, trunk, and pelvis fall in a straight line.

Sitting posture

When we sit in a chair, our hips should be as far back in the chair as possible. Head, spinal column, shoulder and hips should be in straight be in straight line and erect. Legs should touch the ground and not in hanged position. Thighs should be in horizontal position. While we read, the book should be on the table but not too far away or near the eyes. The approximate distance between book and eyes should be at least 30cms. For writing, a table with slight inclination towards outside is appropriate.

Posture of walking

Correct walking is always commended everywhere and by everyone. It reflects the personality of an individual. It indicates inferiority complex if an individual walks with dropped neck and imbalanced steps. If someone walks with erect neck and chest out, it is an example of superiority complex. In fact, the best posture of walking is that, the lines of the feet should be parallel to the line of direction. The heels of the feet should touch the ground and then weight should be transferred to the toes. It means, there should be heel-toe action. Walking should be efficient and graceful. Smoothness is essential in walking. If we adopt wrong posture of walking, we may get fatigue at earliest.

Lying Posture

Normal size of pillow should be used by the children. Hard bed is beneficial for those, who have spinal problems and should sleep in a state where he does not feel any difficulty in respiration.

Importance of good posture in development of personality:

- Appearance
- Grace and efficiency of movements
- Physical fitness
- Hygienic value
- Social value
- Economic value
- Prevents diseases
- Change in mental attitude

Causes of posture deformities:

- Gravitational factors
- Improper diet
- Diseases
- Birth
- Accidents
- Fatigue
- Fashion
- Delicacy and limitation
- Lack of fresh air and light
- Lack of rest and sleep
- Lack of proper exercise
- Lack of awareness
- Unsuitable furniture
- Improve way of carrying weight
- Others reasons

Postural deformities and their remedial measures:

Spinal Curvature: This type of deformity is related to spine. These are of three types:

Kyphosis

It implies an increase or exaggeration of a backward or posterior curve or a decrease or reversal of a forward curve. It is also called round upper back. Depression of chest is common in kyphosis. Kyphosis is caused by malnutrition, illness, crowd, deficient ventilation, insufficient exercise, rickets, carrying heavy loads on shoulders, unsuitable furniture etc. Coach, trainer, teachers, parents may play a vital role in the prevention of this deformity. Students should be taught, how to stand, how to sit and how to walk so that they could adopt good postures. Proper set of exercises can prevent and control the bad posture.

Lordosis

It is the extreme limit of round shoulders. It is an increased forward curve in the lumber region. In this deformity, upper body leans forward. Generally, malnutrition, unhealthy environment, under-development muscles and heavy loads are the main causes of lordosis. Lordosis may be prevented or controlled by same means as that of kyphosis. Curative exercises and habit of accurate posture may be helpful.

Scoliosis

Postural adaptation of the spine in lateral direction is called scoliosis. It means bending, twisting or rotating. In fact, these are sideways curves and may be called scoliotic curves. These are defined in terms of their convexities. They are identified, as either convexities. A simple or single curve to the left or convexity left is commonly called a "c" curve. Scoliotic curves are usually found in "s" shape.

The main reasons of scoliosis are diseases in the joints of bones, underdevelopment legs infantile paralysis, rickets etc. It may also be due to carrying heavy loads on one shoulder, unhealthy conditions like inadequate lighting arrangement, unsuitable desks, partial deafness and wrong standing posture.

Scoliosis may be prevented by having the subject bent forward from the waist with the arms hanging down. This position is called the Adam's position. Hanging by hands is also a good exercise; scoliosis may be controlled by the expert doctor by employing the 'derotation principle' which is a set of exercises involving rotating the thoracic spine in the direction opposite to its assumed position. For example, in case of a dorsal left scoliosis, derotation exercises will involve rotation of the vertebrate to the left.

Knock knees

In this, both knees join together. Feet remain parallel apart when the child stands. The gap between ankles is enhanced. The child feels problem in walking and running. He loses his normal gait. It is caused by rickets and due to the deficiency of calcium and vitamin-D. It may also be due to chronic illness, obesity, flat foot and heavy body weight.

Cod liver oil may be helpful in reducing the deficiency of vitamin-D. Horse riding is the best exercise to control this deformity. Along these, walking calipers may be beneficial. In severe state, doctor should be consulted.

Flat foot

The feet function as the base of support for the body in standing, walking, running and jumping. It is easy to observe whether a person has flat foot or not. He should dip his feet in the water and then he should walk on the floor. If there is not proper arch of the foot prints then that person has flat foot. In fact, there should be a proper arch of the foot. Such persons do not have enough jumping or running ability.

Main cause of flat foot is weak muscles of the foot which cannot bear the body weight. Hence, feet become flat or without arches. Along with this rapid increase in body weight, heavy shoes, carrying heavy weight for a longer period are also the causes of flat foot.

To remove or control this deficiency, shoes with good arches may be used. One should walk on the outward side of the foot. Heavy weight should be avoided. High heeled shoes should also be avoided.

Bow legs

'Bow legs' is also a postural deformity opposite to knock-knees position. If the knees do not touch when standing with feet together, the individual has bow legs or genu varum. In this deformity knees are widely apart. There remains a gap between knees, when a bow legged keeps his feet together. This deformity can be observed easily, when an individual walks or runs.

Main cause of bow legs is the deficiency of calcium and phosphorous in the bones. Long bones of the legs become soft, hence they are bent outward. Bow legs may be due to improper weight bearing or continuous weight bearing. Improper way of walking may also result in bow legs. Bow legs can be prevented by taking balanced diet. In fact, there should not be any deficiency of calcium and phosphorous.

Excessive fatty diet should not be given to the young ones. Young ones should not be forced to walk at early stage. Bow legs can be controlled by walking on the inner edge of feet.

TEST AND EVALUATION

Test

Performance in any sporting event is the result of a multitude of factors, which include the amount of training performed, the body's adaptation to the training, motivation level, nutritional status and weather conditions to name a few. As you can see, physiological parameters only account for a portion of any performance, and so the role of any exercise physiologist is also similarly limited. Through fitness testing, the factors involving physiological processes, over which there is some control, can be measured and ultimately improved upon. Competition is the ultimate test of performance capability, and is therefore the best indication of training success. Fitness testing attempts to measure individual components of performance, with the ultimate aim of studying and maximizing the athlete's ability in each component.

Benefits of Test

To identify weaknesses and strengths is the one benefit of fitness testing. The major use is to establish the strengths and weaknesses of the athlete. This is done by comparing test results to other athletes in the same training group, the same sport, or a similar population group. Previous test results of large groups are often published as normative tables. By comparing results to successful athletes in your sport, you can see the areas which need improvement, and the training program can be modified accordingly. This way valuable training time can be used more efficiently. However, beware that some athletes perform well in their sport despite their physical or physiological attributes, and it may not be advantageous to be like them.

Safety

Safety checks should be done prior to any testing session, such as checking for the proper working of equipment, and adequate supply of safety equipment such as mats, water bottles and first aid kits. During the sessions, give adequate warm-up when necessary (see more about warming up for fitness testing). For maximal endurance testing on elderly and special populations (after medical clearance has been given), medical assistance should be close at hand, and adequate resuscitation equipment should be available nearby.

Any person older than thirty five years of age, particularly anyone overweight or with a history of high blood pressure and heart disease should consult a physician before undertaking any vigorous testing. Fitness testing should not be avoided, as for this population it can be useful as a screening device and to help devise a program to suit special needs. For all participants that are not accustomed to exercise, it would be wise to conduct a PARQ – Physical Activity Readiness Questionnaire.

Observe Progress

The initial testing session can give the athlete an idea of where their fitness levels are at the start of a program, so that future testing can be compared to this and any changes can be noted. A baseline is especially important if you are about to get on a new training phase. Subsequent tests should be planned for the end and start of each new phase.

By repeating tests at regular intervals, you can get an idea of the effectiveness of the training program, the time frame between tests can depend on the availability of time or costs involved, or the phase of training the athlete is in. Depending on these factors, the period between tests may range from four weeks to eight months. It usually takes a minimum of 4–8 weeks to see a demonstrable change in any aspect of fitness.

Talent detection

Testing is primarily used for help in designing the most appropriate athletic training program. A general non-sport specific testing battery can provide you with an idea of your basic strengths and weaknesses, and from this you may find you would be better suited to which another sport which makes better use of your strengths. Although testing has sometimes been used in this way for talent identification, it has generally not been very reliable in predicting the future success of juniors and in sports which rely heavily on other factors such as technique, tactics and psychological factors.

Selecting Test

There is often a standard set of tests that are performed for the fitness testing of any sport. If you do not have access to such list or you wish to modify a protocol to suit individual needs, you can use the following information to design your own testing regime. Remember that the fitness test that best determines your capability in any component of fitness is not always the most appropriate test to perform; there are many other factors to consider.

Identifying Components of Performance

The first step in designing a fitness testing regimen is to identify the components of fitness that you wish to investigate. These may depend on the phase of training or the phase of the season in which the testing is being done. Each sport requires certain attributes and relies on certain factors more than others for successful performance.

Example: You would not necessarily want to test a marathon runner on sprinting speed. Your fitness testing time could be better spent on doing more relevant tests. One method of categorizing the different components of fitness are as presented on the list of tests, though this categorization is somewhat random. Your testing sequence may include a few similar tests from one fitness component and none from others, depending on what your aims of the testing are.

Standardized Protocols

The test reports need to be standardized so that comparisons can be made between your test scores performed at different times and comparisons between athletes tested at different places. Athletes and coaches should be aware of the need to control the factors which can affect the results obtained. Such things that need to be controlled are:

- The warm up
- Order of tests
- Recovery periods

- Environmental conditions
- Fluid
- Nutritional status

If comparing test results to normative tables, the test must be conducted exactly the same as it was when the original test group was tested, for the comparison to be valid.

Significance

You need to select sport specific tests. If you believe that the tests are significant to the sport you play, you will be more inclined to put a maximal effort into the testing. If not, you can be wasting valuable time on tests that are not significant to your particular sport, and the results will be meaningless.

Reliability

A test is considered reliable if the results are consistent and re-producible over time. You should be able to obtain the same or similar result on three separate trials. This is important as you are often looking for small changes in scores, and you want the difference in results to reflect the changes in fitness of the person and not an error in measurement. Some of the errors in recording of test's results can come about from poor following of the test protocols, equipment error or variability in environmental conditions. Reliability can be improved by greater control of these variables, and by using competent and well trained testers, though there is still some variability expected. All the equipments used should be standard and regularly calibrated to the manufacturer's standards. If more than one test is being conducted at a time, the ordering of tests can affect results for each test, as can be training and fatigue of the athlete between test sessions. If the test requires pacing or practice, the more experienced athletes will do better at maximizing their performance and their score will be more reliable.

Validity

Validity is whether the tests actually measure what they set out to be measure. It is quite possible that a test can be very reliable but not valid. The validity of a test is usually better if the test is specific to the sport being tested or the tests should resemble the sport being tested, so that similar actions and therefore the specific muscle groups and muscle fiber types actually used in the sport are being used. There are different forms of validity:

- Internal
- External
- Ecological

For an experiment to possess ecological validity, the methods, materials and setting of the experiment must approximate the real life situation that is under study. A fitness test having external and ecological validity enables you to make generalization about their sports performance from specific tests.

Facilities and Other Demands

The time, cost, equipment and personnel required can be the most important considerations while selecting a test, and often determines what tests are actually conducted. This is especially important if you intend to test large groups of athletes.

Interpretable Results

If you don't know what the numbers in the results mean, the tests are fairly useless. The results must have meaning so that they can be applied to modify a training program. If you want to compare the results to that of other groups you must have access to normative data ('norms'). These norms should be based on a large homogeneous population, be up to date, and preferably be of local origin.

Conducting Test

Test groundwork

To ensure that each subject is primed physically to perform up to their potential, they should follow set nutritional and physical guidelines. If all participants follow the same procedures and are in the same physical state, then comparisons are more valid and if the same procedures are followed for each testing session, then the results will be more reliable.

Test Sequence

The order in which the fitness tests are performed can affect the performance in subsequent tests. Here are some guidelines while deciding in which order to conduct the test. These are guidelines that can be used to determine the best order in your situation. There are other factors to consider such as logistics of getting from one test location to another, group sizes, number of assessor, and time constraints. Whatever order is used should be recorded made consistent for future testing sessions.

Health Checks: Blood pressure and resting heart rate should always be tested first while the person is fully relaxed.

Anthropometry: There should be no physical activity prior to the measurements of body composition. This test should always be done firstly and directly after any health checks.

Flexibility: Depending on whether the test protocol requires a warm up or not, the flexibility tests should be scheduled early in the session prior to any activity or after a thorough warm up or after the speed tests.

Speed/Power tests: Power tests are usually performed first, followed by speed, agility, strength, muscle endurance and finally cardio respiratory or repeat sprint tests. A thorough warm-up should precede any speed and power test. The vertical jump test may be performed prior to the sprint test.

Muscle Strength: Muscle strength (1–10RM) tests should always be completed prior to muscle endurance tests, but after the speed and power tests.

Muscular Endurance: A minimum break of five minutes is recommended between muscle strength and muscle endurance tests. If there are several muscular strength and endurance tests in one session, you must allow plenty of time for recovery between tests.

Aerobic Fitness: Many of the sub maximal aerobic tests are based on a heart rate response may be affected by previous tests and by the mental state of the athlete, and should be scheduled accordingly. Fatigue maximal exercise tests, such as a VO_2max or beep test and repeat sprint tests, should always be scheduled at the end of a session. If the protocol includes both a repeat sprint test and a maximal aerobic test, it is usually wise to have these in separate sessions.

Scheduling

Testing should be done at particular times that correspond to the aims of the tests. For example, you may wish to test at the beginning of certain phases of training and then at regular intervals to monitor progress. For school groups it may be appropriate to schedule testing at the beginning and ends of school semesters.

Recording Sheets

Well-designed scoring sheets should be used for recording scores to be more efficient and avoiding errors. Those should include space for all relevant information. In addition to the test results, the following should also be recorded with every testing session:

Test Assistants

All test assistants should be adequately trained prior to testing, to ensure correct administration of the tests, and reduce error between tests.

Session Organization

Good organization will ensure that the testing session runs smoothly. If testing a large group, you may want to set up testing stations with a different tester at each station, or with one tester following the same group around the stations.

Interpretation of Results

Relative Importance

The first step in the interpretation of test results requires you to determine how important each of the components that were tested is to the overall performance in the sport. For example, while a poor result in a body fat test for a basketball player may be of concern, it is not as vital as a poor result in an endurance test. The relative importance of each fitness component normally requires a good understanding of the physiology involved, and so is best done by a qualified exercise physiologist.

Comparison to Norms

If the results are being compared to normative values (norms), you must consider if the norms used the same protocol, and the subject population and age group are similar. Also, published norms and rating charts may give the averages for a certain population, but this does not always indicate what the desirable level for that particular parameter is fitness norms.

Significance

Are the changes seen from test to test significant? There is normal variation in results from test to test due to factors such as biological variation, tester error, equipment calibrations, conditions, etc. So, one must decide if the differences recorded are significant to affect performance and are greater than expected from general sources of error.

Requirements

- To undertake this test you will require:
- Flat non-slip surface
- Mat
- Stopwatch
- Assistant

How to conduct the test

The assistant is responsible for instructing the athlete as to the position to assume at the appropriate stage. Throughout the test the back, neck and head should be maintained in the posture as per figure below. If the athlete is unable to hold this position then the test is to be stopped.

Stage 1

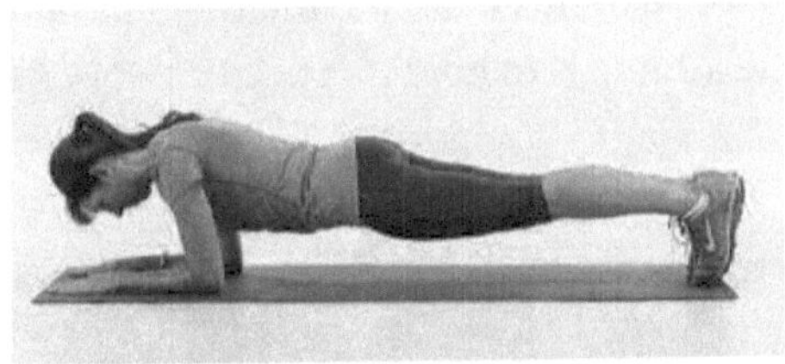

The athlete warms up for 10 minutes

The athlete while using the mat to support their elbows and arms assumes the Start Position Once the athlete is in the correct position. The assistant starts the stopwatch. The athlete is to hold this position for 60 seconds.

Stage 2

The athlete lifts their right arm off the ground and extends it out in front of them parallel with the ground. The athlete is to hold this position for 15 seconds.

Stage 3

The athlete returns to the Start Position, lifts the left arm off the ground and extends it out in front of them parallel with the ground. The athlete is to hold this position for 15 seconds.

Stage 4

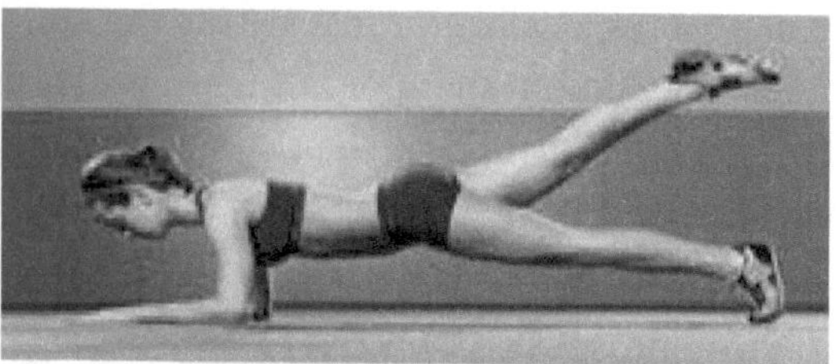

The athlete returns to the Start Position, lifts the right leg off the ground and extends it out behind them parallel with the ground. The athlete is to hold this position for 15 seconds.

Stage 5

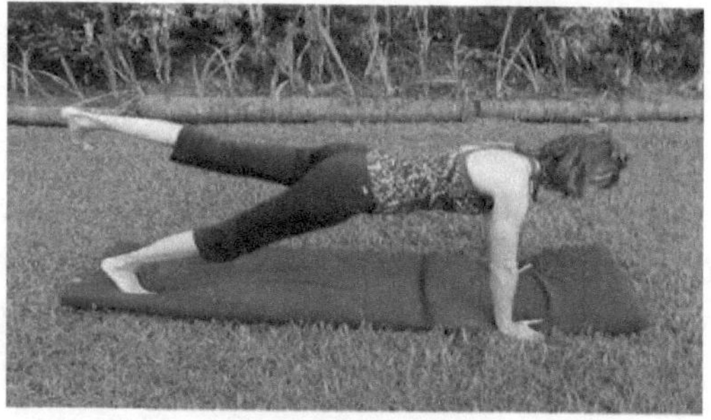

The athlete returns to the Start Position, lifts the left leg off the ground and extends it out behind them parallel with the ground. The athlete is to hold this position for 15 seconds.

Stage 6

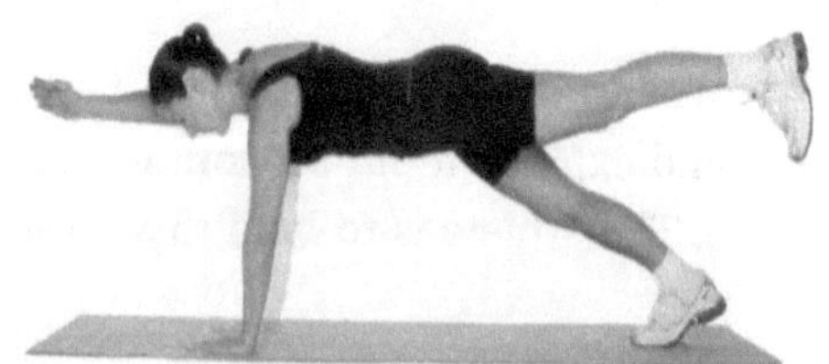

The athlete returns to the Start Position, lifts the left leg and right arm off the ground and extends them out parallel with the ground. The athlete is to hold this position for 15 seconds.

Stage 7

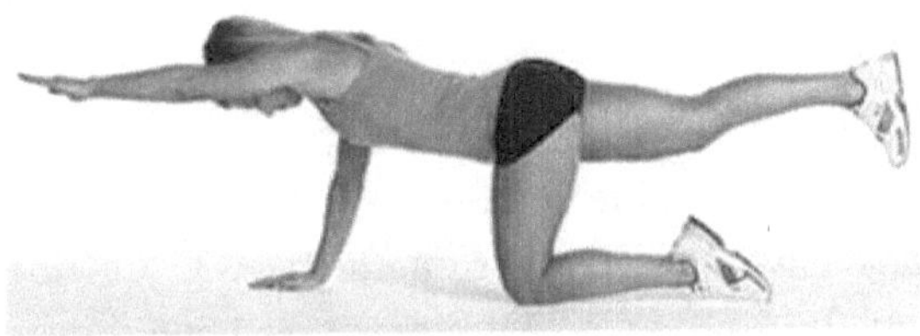

The athlete returns to the Start Position, lifts the right leg and left arm off the ground and extends them out parallel with the ground. The athlete is to hold this position for 15 seconds.

Stage 8

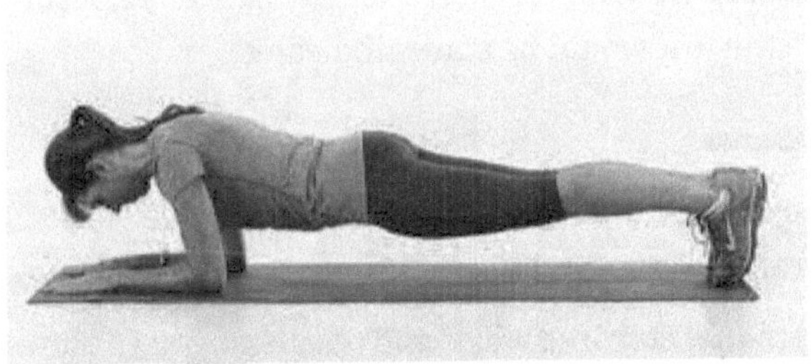

The athlete returns to the Start Position. The athlete is to hold this position for 30 seconds.

End of Test

The assistant records the stage at which the athlete is unable to maintain the correct body position or is unable to continue with the test.

Analysis

Analysis of the result is by comparing it with the results of previous tests. It is expected that, with appropriate training between each test, the analysis would indicate an improvement.

If the athlete is able to complete this test then it indicates that they have good core strength. If they are unable to complete the test then repeat the routine 3 or 4 times a week until they are able to complete. If core strength is poor then the torso will move unnecessarily during motion and waste energy. Good core strength indicates that the athlete can move with high efficiency.

Target Group

This test is suitable for active individuals but not for those where the test would be contraindicated.

Side Ramp

Purpose: The side ramp test measures the control and endurance of the lateral core stabilizing muscles.

Equipment required: flat and clean surface, stopwatch, recording sheets and pen.

Procedure: The aim of this test is to hold an elevated position for as long as possible. The subject lays on their right side; the upper body is supported off the ground by the right elbow and forearm. The legs are straight, with the left foot (top) in front of your right foot. The hip is lifted off the floor so that the elbow and feet support the body, creating a straight line from head to toe. The left hand is placed on the supporting shoulder. As soon as the subject is in the correct position, the stopwatch is started. The test is over when the subject is unable to hold the back straight and the hip is lowered. After five minutes rest, the other side is tested.

Scoring: The score is the total time completed for each side. Compare the performance on the two sides. The table below indicates guideline rating scores for both males and females.

Rating	Time (seconds)
Excellent	> 90
Good	75 to 90
Average	60 to 75
Poor	< 60

Test Leg Raises

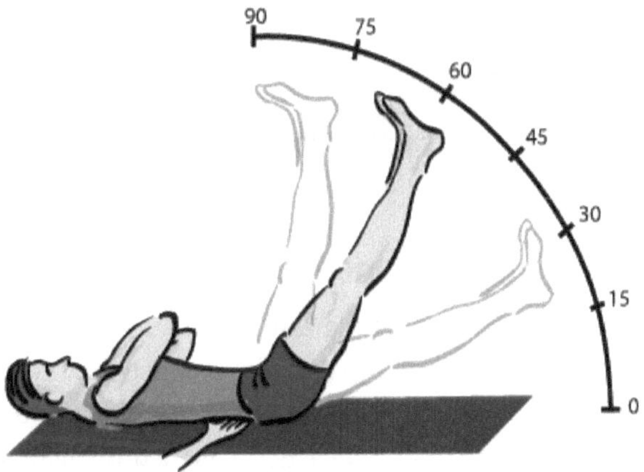

The Leg Raise Test measures core stability by completing as many leg raises as possible while supporting body weight, all in time to a beep recording. This test was used in testing for Australia's Greatest Athlete, and called the Diving Challenge.

Purpose: The leg raise test measures the control and endurance of the core stabilizing muscles.

Equipment required: leg raise machine, metronome or cadence recording. A beep recording can be created using the Team Beep Test software.

Procedure: The aim of this test is to perform as many leg lifts as possible, in time to recorded beeps. The subjects start in the leg raise machine, with their weight supported on their elbows and forearm and legs hanging down. When ready, the metronome or beeps are started. The subject must raise the legs (keeping the knees straight) to a horizontal position and then back again. The test is over when the subject is unable to perform the action correctly in time to the beeps.

Scoring: The score is the maximum number of complete repetitions successfully performed.

Abdominal Strength

In the abdominal strength test is measure the ability of the abdominal muscle.

Abdominal Endurance

In the abdominal endurance test is measure the ability to perform repeated abdominal curls in a set time (e.g. one minute) or at a set rate. What test you use will be dependent of what you are trying to measure, weighed up against the costs and ease of conducting the test.

The techniques for the abdominal endurance sit-up tests are used for the US defense forces (US Army, US Marines, and US Navy), the home test and other endurance tests vary slightly. Make note of the instructions such as where the hands are held (across the chest, behind the head, on the side of the head, out in front), how far you have to go back (shoulders to the ground, head to touch) and how far you go up (to touch your knees, chest to thighs), the angle of the knees (usually 90 degrees) and whether the feet are held or not. Being consistent with the technique will improve the reliability of the tests. When comparing the results to normative values, you should make sure that the testing techniques, test conditions and subject populations are the same.

Sit Up Endurance Tests: are usually conducted over a one minute period, and measure the maximum number of correctly performed sit-ups in that time. The home test is one example of this. The Army, Navy and Marines use a two minute test, and allow rest breaks. An alternative to the one or two minute test is a sit-up test that is continued until exhaustion at a given pace given by a metronome or audio recording.

Sit Up Strength Tests: do not require repeated sit-ups to be performed. The 7-Stage and the simpler variation the 4-Level test require the subject to perform sit ups of increasing difficulty. Similarly, the Straight Leg Lift monitors the ability of the abdominal muscles to function as the difficulty of the movement increases.

Seven Stage Abdominal Strength Test

This is an easy way to perform sit up test of abdominal strength that can be done with large groups all at once.

Purpose: The 8-level sit up test measures abdominal strength, which is important in back support and core stability.

Equipment required: flat surface, 5 lb (2.5 kg) and 10 lb (5 kg) weight, recording sheet and pen.

Procedure: The subject lies on their back, with their knees at right angles and feet flat on the floor, the subject then attempts to perform one complete sit-up for each level in the prescribed manner (see table below), starting with level 1. Each level is achieved if a single sit up is performed in the prescribed manner, without the feet coming off the floor. As many attempts as necessary can be made.

Scoring: There are 8 levels ranging in difficulty from very poor to elite. The highest level sit-up correctly completed is recorded.

Level	Rating	Description
0	very poor	cannot perform level 1
1	poor	with arms extended, the athlete curls up so that the wrists reach the knees
2	fair	with arms extended, the athlete curls up so that the elbows reach the knees
3	average	with the arms held together across abdominals, the athletes curls up so that the chest touches the thighs
4	good	with the arms held across chest, holding the opposite shoulders, the athlete curls up so that the forearms touch the thighs
5	very good	with the hands held behind head, the athlete curls up so that the chest touches the thighs

Level	Rating	Description
6	excellent	as per level 5, with a 5 lb (2.5 kg) weight held behind head, chest touching the thighs
7	elite	as per level 5, with a 10 lb (5 kg) weight held behind head, chest touching the thighs

List of Other Tests

- 7-Stage Abdominal Strength Test
- 4-Level Abdominal Strength Test
- Straight Leg Abdominal Strength Test
- Abdominal Endurance Tests
- Curl Ups (President's Challenge)
- Partial Curl Ups
- NCF Abdominal Curl Conditioning Test
- Home Sit Up Test
- US Army Sit Up Test
- US Marines Sit Up Test
- US Navy Sit Up Test
- Euro fit 30sec Sit Up Test

APFT Sit up Test

This abdominal muscle fitness test forms part of the Army Physical Fitness Test (APFT) is performed by US Army personnel after every six months.

Purpose: This test measures the endurance of the abdominal and hip-flexor muscles.

Equipment required: Floor mat or flat ground, stopwatch

Procedure: The aim of this test is to perform as many sit-ups as you can do in two minutes. The starting position is lying on your back with your knees bent at a 90-degree angle. Feet may be up to 12 inches apart. Your fingers must be interlocked behind your head. A second person holds your ankles with the hands only. On the command 'get set,' the starting position is assumed, and on the command 'go,' start the sit-up by raising your upper body forward to or beyond the vertical position (meaning that the base of your neck is above the base of your spine), and then lower your body until the bottom of your shoulder blades and the backs of your hands touch the ground. Pausing to rest is permitted only in the up position.

Scoring: The maximum number of correctly performed sit ups is recorded. The scoring depends on the sex and age of the participant.

Comments: The sit up will not be counted if you fail to reach the vertical position, fail to keep your fingers interlocked behind your head, arch or bow your back and raise your buttocks off the ground to raise your upper body, or let your knees exceed a 90-degree angle. The heel is the only part of your foot that must stay in contact with the ground. Your head, hands, arms, or elbows do not have to touch the ground.There are many exercises available for developing strong abs and building core strength, but few methods offered for evaluating that strength. Sports Coach, Brian Mackenzie offers the following Core Muscle Strength and Stability Test as a way to determine your current core strength and gauge your progress over time.

The Core Muscle Strength & Stability Test

The objective of this evaluation is to monitor the development and improvements of an athlete's core strength and endurance over time. To prepare for the assessment you will need:

- Flat surface
- Mat
- Watch or clock with second counter

Conducting the Test

- Position the watch or clock where you can easily see it.
- Start in the Plank Exercise Position (elbows on the ground) Hold for 60 seconds.
- Lift your right arm off the ground stop for 15 seconds.
- Return your right arm to the ground and lift the left arm off the ground Hold for 15 seconds.
- Return your left arm to the ground and lift the right leg off the ground Hold for 15 seconds.
- Return your right leg to the ground and lift the left leg off the ground Hold for 15 seconds.
- Lift your left leg and right arm off the ground Hold for 15 seconds
- Return your left leg and right arm to the ground.
- Lift your right leg and left arm off the ground Hold for 15 seconds.
- Return to the Plank Exercise Position (elbows on the ground) Hold this position for 30 seconds.

Results

Good Core Strength

If you can complete the test fully, you have good core strength.

Poor Core Strength

If one cannot complete the test fully, it indicates that the core strength needs improvement. Poor core strength results in unnecessary torso movement and swaying during all other athletic movements resulting in wasted energy and poor biomechanics. Good core strength indicates that the athlete can move with high efficiency. If one is unable to complete the test, then one should doing it. By comparing one's results over time, one will note improvements or decline in core strength.

YOUNG ATHLETES

As per National Strength and Conditioning Association Education Department, more coaches and parents are asking the question, "When is it safe for my child to start strength training?" Several other questions, such as "What exercises should young athletes perform?" and "How often should they engage in strength training?" This chapter is designed to shed some light on these, and other questions and dispel some common 'myths' surrounding youth strength training.

Let's define some terms So that we are all on the same page, it is important that we define some common terms that will be used throughout this chapter. The National Strength and Conditioning Association (NSCA) define youth as a child who has not yet reached, or is going through, physical maturity. Recognize that not all children progress through puberty at the same time or at the same rate. Three athletes of the same chronological age (i.e. all are 12 years old) can differ by ± two years in biological age. Even though you have three athletes of twelve year olds, maturity wise they can range in age from 10–14. Strength training is synonymous with the term 'resistance training' and is defined as a specialized form of conditioning that is used to increase one's ability to produce or resist force. Strength training uses the principle of progressive overload to force the body to adapt in order to be able to produce and or resist larger forces.

Strength training is not power lifting nor is it bodybuilding or trying to lift the most weight you can. Strength training is a tool that can augment sport performance through improved strength and motor control. Is youth strength training safe? The risk of injury is probably the primary concern of any coach or parent who has a child beginning a strength training program. Any exercise or activity carries with it some risk of injury even when a child is running in the backyard can suffer with an injury. It is unrealistic, therefore, to assume that injuries will never occur. However, this risk of injury can be minimized substantially by following a few simple guidelines. Specifically, appropriate training and competent supervision are the two keys to minimizing all injuries. Both the NSCA and the American Academy of Pediatrics state that youth strength training can be safe and effective if:

A competent coach who is skilled in program design supervises every strength training session. Proper technique is taught and required. Even with this information, several safety concerns still exist. Two of the most common concerns raised by the parents and coaches are addressed below.

Two of the most common concerns raised by the parents and coaches are, about the damages the growth of plates and overuse/soft-tissue injuries, are addressed below.

Concern #1

Do strength training damage growth plates in bones?

Most parents and coaches are hesitant to begin strength training with young athletes due to fear of damaging the bones and possibly stunting growth. Almost everyone has heard a story of some children experiencing stunted growth after damaging a bone's growth plate from lifting weights. This story could be considered as an "urban legend," a story that everyone has heard, but no one knows if it is in fact true. Before going any further, let's define the term growth plate. In children, all bone growth occurs at a region of cartilage near the ends of the bone. This region is weaker than mature bone and may be at a greater risk for injury. If the growth plate is damaged there is a chance that growth in the bone will be stunted. The fact is that no growth plate fractures have been documented in athletes who engage in a resistance training program that includes

"An appropriately prescribed training regimen and competent instruction."

The risk of injury to the growth plates can be further minimized by not allowing the athletes to lift weight over their heads or perform maximum effort lifts. A general rule of thumb when working with younger athletes is to have them only exercise with weights that they can lift six times or more. Growth plate injuries should be taken seriously because they can happen. However, with proper care, the risk can be virtually eliminated.

Concern #2

Do overuse injuries occur with strength training?

The potential for repetitive use injuries to the soft tissue of the body is another concern for young athletes entering a strength training program. These types of injuries do occur. The majority (40–70 %) of strength training related soft-tissue injuries are muscles strains with the lower back being the most frequently injured area. Again, these types of injuries can be minimized by following a few simple guidelines:

- Teach the athletes proper technique for each exercise that is performed,
- Supervise every strength training session,
- Do not have the athletes train with maximal or near-maximal loads,
- Avoid using resistive devices that are supposed to improve vertical jump height,

Benefits of Youth Strength Training

- Improved strength and coordination,
- Increased muscle endurance,
- Improved sport performance,
- Increased bone density,
- Improved heath,
- Improved bone strength bone density,
- Reduced risk for injury,
- Improved self-image and self-confidence.

Concern #3

Does strength training work for your athletes?

Yes, strength training can benefit young athletes. Some of these benefits are highlighted in the accompanying table. Most people believe that testosterone (a steroid produced naturally in the body that plays a role in increased muscle mass and, consequently, increased strength) is necessary to build strength. However, there are also other mechanisms that can produce strength gains. Since young athletes (and female athletes) do not produce large amounts of testosterone there for the mechanism behind the strength gains differs from what is seen in adults. Resistance training helps to improve motor control and "teaching" muscles how to work together in a coordinated manner. Even within a muscle, strength training helps to synchronize the contraction of individual fibers which leads to improvements in strength without gaining any additional muscle mass. Therefore, do not expect a young athlete to develop much new muscle mass when they begin strength training, since testosterone and other hormones that are required for the building of new muscle mass is not present in large quantities.

Designing a Strength Training Program probably the best way to introduce athletes to the wonderful world of strength training is to have them perform 'body-weight' exercises. As you might guess, these exercises use the athlete's own body weight as the resistance. These exercises can include:

- Push Ups, Pull ups, Sit ups, Back extensions, Body weight lunges or squats, Step-ups, and Dips.

The benefits of these exercises are several-fold. First, this type of exercise is inexpensive and easy to implement. Second, these exercises strengthen the core muscles of the body (the core is defined as the muscles surrounding the body's center of mass – namely the abs, lower back, and hip musculature) that help to stabilize the body. It is important to develop a solid strength base in these muscles before progressing on to more advanced exercises. The initial goal of any program should be to build some muscular endurance. Start out slowly, initially performing one set of 15 repetitions. As the athletes develop, strive to complete three sets of each exercise, each containing six-fifteen repetitions, three times and a week as part of the regular program. As an athlete matures physically and emotionally, you can begin to introduce more complex exercises (multi-joint lifts, free weights, and low intensity plyometrics exercises) into the program. However, even the most basic multi-joint exercise requires a solid strength base in the body's core musculature to minimize the risk of injury. If strength training is a part of the overall training program, it is important to make it consistent – when strength training is stopped, detraining (a loss of strength and the strength associated benefits) will occur.

Concern #4

Questions to ask before starting a strength training program, there are several questions you should ask yourself (or the strength coach if that is not you) before embarking on a strength training plan for your young athletes. Is the athlete physically and emotionally mature enough to engage in a strength training program?

As mentioned, you want to start young athletes on a program that centers on muscular endurance and building strength in the core muscles of the body. As an athlete matures, he or she can progress on to more complex exercises, such as multi-joint exercises or lifting free weights. Athletes need to show the maturity, both physical and mental, to advance to these more complex exercises. Keep in mind those athletes of the same chronological age' can differ by as much as ± two years physically or mentally. Also keep in mind that females mature as much as two years earlier than males. If machines or equipments are being used, is it sized appropriately for a young athlete? Most equipment in strength and conditioning facility will be sized to meet the needs of an adult and not a young athlete. Make sure you can adjust any equipment to the size of the child. If you cannot, then do not perform the exercise until the child "grows into" the equipment. When the need arises for "size appropriate" equipment, dumbbells and most free weights can be used.

Dumbbells and free weights allow you to accommodate for differences in the size of the athletes and eliminate the need for purchasing junior/youth equipment.

Concern #5

Is the program going to be properly run and supervised?

Proper supervision and teaching are essential to running a safe and injury-free strength training program. The NSCA recommends a 1:10 coach to athlete ratio for young athletes. Strength training is more than just throwing a bunch of exercises together; a program should be carefully tailored to the needs of the athlete and the sport.

NSCA's Recommendations for Youth Strength Training

- All athletes should be taught proper exercise and spotting technique.
- Exercises should initially be taught with no load to allow proper technique to be learned.
- All training sessions should be supervised by an experienced fitness professional.
- Each child should be physically and emotionally prepared to participate in a strength training program. Also consider the athlete's maturity level when introducing more advanced exercises.

- Children should have realistic expectations or goals.
- The exercise area should be safe and free from hazards.
- Every exercise session should be preceded by approximately five-ten minutes of a general warm-up, followed by several sport specific warm-up exercises performed at a light intensity.
- Equipment should be properly sized for a child.
- Begin lifting, preferably, with body weight exercises. Athletes can also be engaged in basic machine exercises if they use light loads that allow the athlete to complete twelve-fifteen repetitions.
- The program should progress to ultimately encourage athletes to perform one-three sets of the exercises on two-three non-consecutive days. Each set should consist of six-fifteen repetitions.
- Never increase the load being lifted by more than five percent for upper body or 10% for lower body exercises.
- Competition between children should be discouraged since this may lead to athletes performing maximum lifts.
- Strength training should be stopped at any sign of injury and the child should be evaluated prior to re-entering the strength program.
- Never force a child to participate in a resistance-training program.
- Keep the program fun.

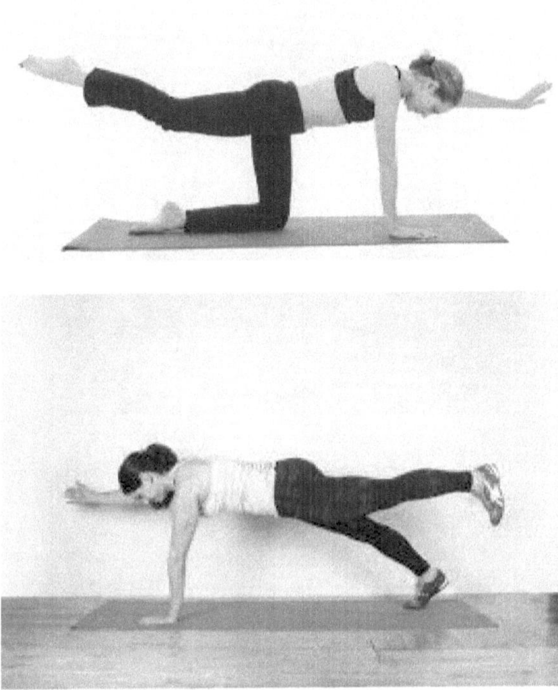

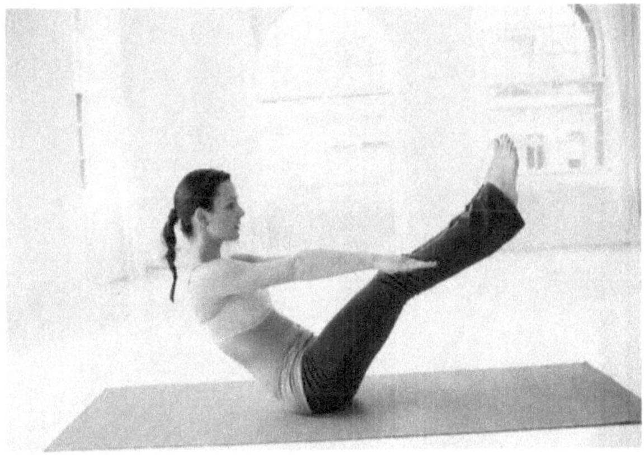

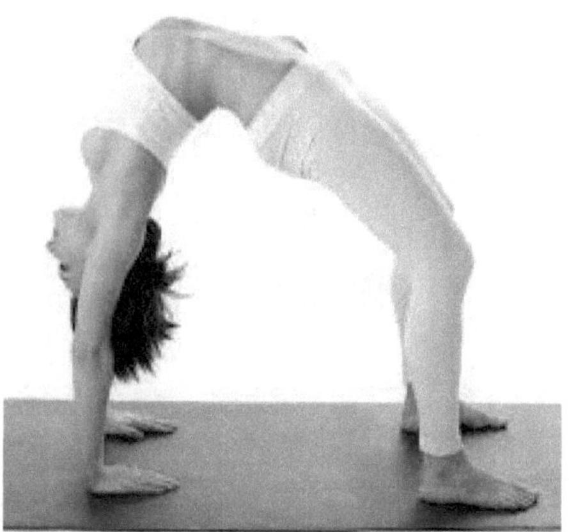

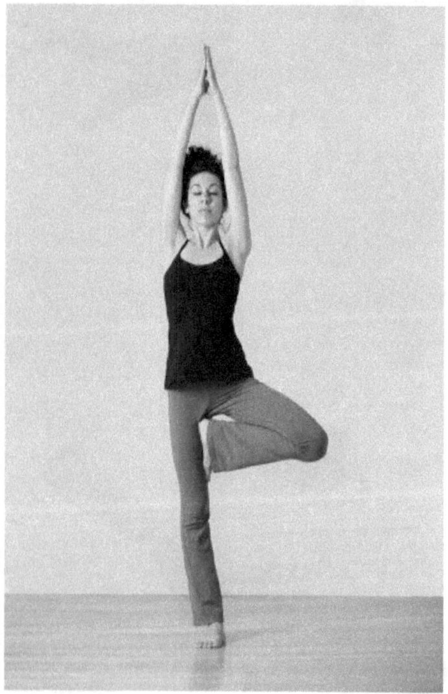

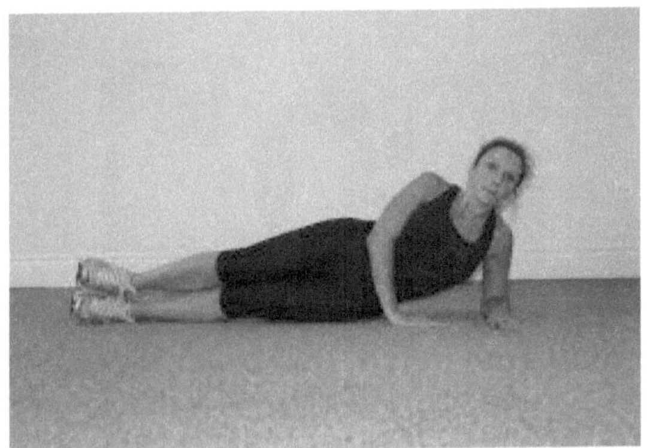

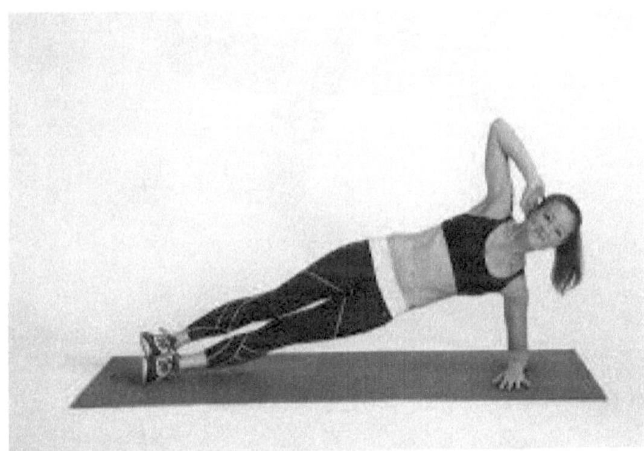

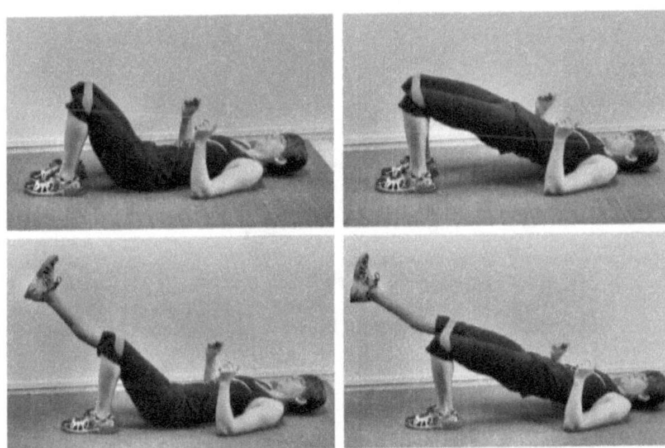

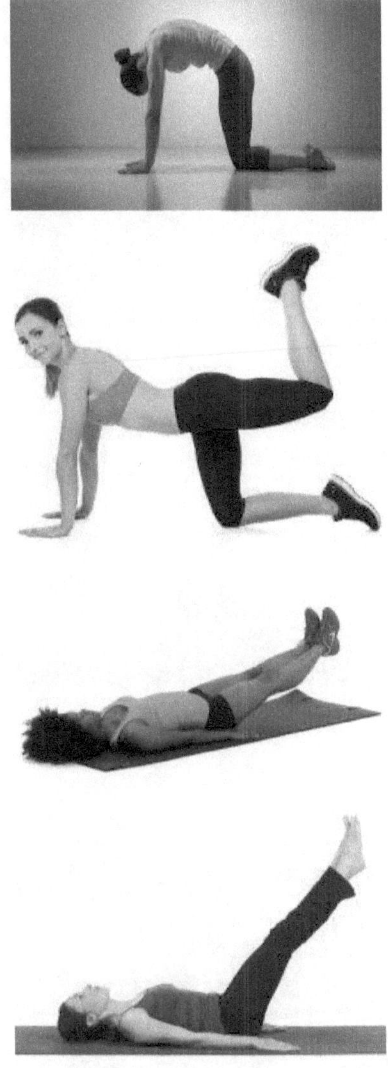

OLDER ADULTS

Exercise

While the continuation of relatively high levels of intellectual activity is linked with the maintenance of cognitive skills in older age, exercise is important to maintain physical fitness of the body as we grow older. Exercise keeps some lifestyle-associated diseases at bay, such as osteoporosis (softening of the bones), heart disease and type II diabetes. In short, 'Use it or lose it'! Exercise has a positive effect on all systems of the body including heart-lung performance, muscular-skeletal activity, neuronal efficiency and body composition. With exercise, the heart muscle strengthens, allowing the heart to pump a larger volume of blood with each beat. This helps to reduce resting blood pressure. Regular aerobic exercise is exercise that can be carried out continuously at a sustained rate.

Therefore, if the lungs are ageing but regularly exercised, they are more likely to retain their function. By strengthening large muscle groups we improve our ability to perform in reflex contractions and muscle endurance. Improving bone strength provides better support for the body, and better posture which in itself reduces the potential for injury. Weight bearing exercise helps to keep bones strong and reduces the risk of osteoporosis. Exercise promotes better neuromuscular (nervous control) function. As we age it is important to maintain our Central Nervous

Control for balance and skilled movement. Lastly our body composition or physical appearance is not only a health issue but also a self esteem one. Our body size and shape can affect how we feel about ourselves, no matter what age we are. Therefore, the benefit of exercise is not only physical (actual body size) but also encompasses physiological and psychological well-being. Aches and pains together with an increase in disease conditions were once considered as a part of 'just getting old. While ageing is characterized by a steady decline in functionality of the various body systems, exercise can reduce this functional decline. It is now believed that much so called 'inevitable ageing' is brought on by inactivity and disuse rather than the ageing process itself.

A major concern associated with ageing is the increased risk of falls as we get older, which sometimes lead to fracture. Fractures can alter mobility for an extended period of time, even indefinitely. Whether falls occur from an uneven footpath, wet shopping mall surface or tripping down stairs, these accidents can sometimes be avoided with better physical conditioning. According Nutrition Fact Sheet it's never too late to Start an Exercise Program Simple exercises that enhance strength, balance, core stability and general aerobic.

Fitness can have a great effect on reducing your chances of a fall. The structure and functions of the body are critical in assisting the older adult to minimize the risk of falling. An exercise program adapted to reduce this risk would include:

- Strength Training
- General fitness
- Aerobic Fitness
- Core Stability

- Balance and Coordination
- Strength Training

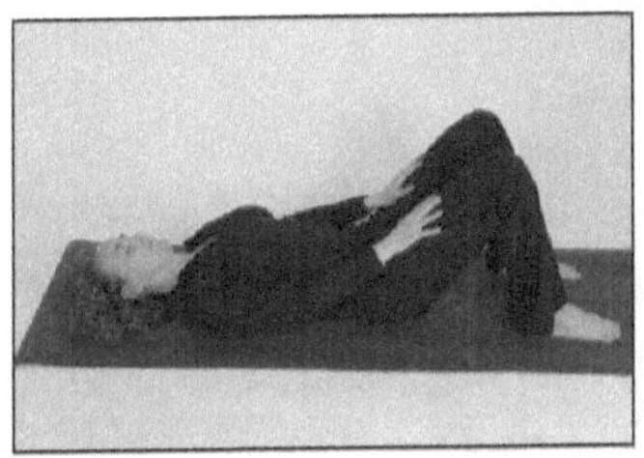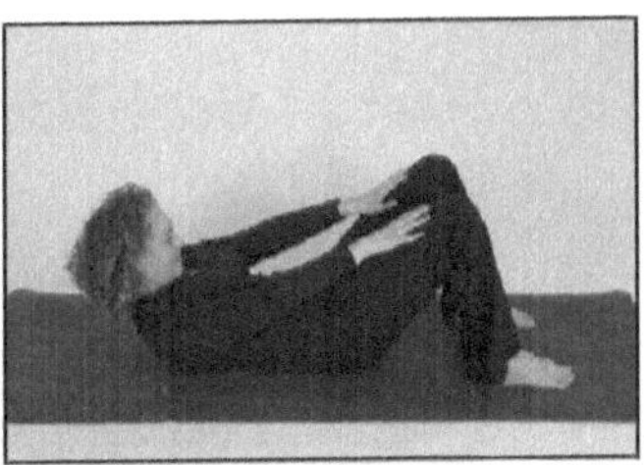

The focus here should be on the legs and abdomen. Most people fall from a standing position, so strong agile legs which are slow to fatigue are best for supporting the body and preventing a fall from occurring. The stomach muscles act like a corset around the spine, and strong deep stomach muscles will help to give support the back. Functional exercises like squats, lunges, and step ups are great for increasing strength. Using weight machines at a gym is not always the best idea as they do not provide multi-directional movement similar to what we perform in daily activity. Abdominal sit ups and stomach crunches are good external stomach exercises but it is really important to also strengthen the deep 'corset' spinal supporting muscles. For this kind of strengthening, classes in yoga or Pilates or a few sessions with a trained professional is a great investment.

General/Aerobic Fitness

A simple free activity such as walking can help reduce the risk of falling simply by increasing the amount of time spent on 'training' the feet in a controlled fatigued state. People who exercise regularly generally get tired at a slower rate. Falling can occur for the simplest reason, such as being too tired to lift your feet high enough to take another step. People who exercise also have a greater awareness of the environment, which in itself decreases the chances of a fall.

Main Part of Core Stability

Core stability means having balance from the 'core' or trunk of the body. The trunk (torso) is like the powerhouse (strength), or should be, the powerhouse of the body. So many people of all ages who attend gyms very often strengthen their body from the 'outside-in' rather than from the 'inside-out.' When liftweights (plates) to achieve big strong arms and legs, it's important to be aware of the extra stress that these heavier appendages might transfer to on torso.

It is equally important to strengthen the deep abdominal muscles which aid in spinal stability. After all, it is the spine that holds the weight of the body upright. Every time you move your body, it tends to sway in the direction of movement until sub-conscious muscle control returns the body back to its normal position. For example, as you walk, you are exposing your body to a series of 'falling over's' in a forward direction. Someone with good core stability has the ability to control this.

Natural body sway, Good core stability strongly relates to good balance and good posture. You don't need to go to a gym to perform Core Stability exercises. They can be done in a chair, lying on the floor or using a fit ball. Yoga and Pilates are good ways to learn exercises for core stability. Having a few sessions with a physiotherapist or exercise professional would be very useful. It's always a good idea to seek professional advice when using a fit ball to make sure it is being used correctly.

Balance

Balance involves brain-muscle coordination, which is essential when trying to prevent falls. It is very important to obtain professional assistance when starting a specific balance program that will ensure initial supervision. Obviously, the worst thing you could do is have a fall when you begin a balance program! Balance is a highly trainable physical characteristic which can often improve rapidly.

Many professional athletes include sport specific balancing programs to improve performance. Variety is the key, the more you vary your exercise routine the more chance you have of exercising different muscles and joints. It is great to take up opportunities of all types of exercise to keep the body and mind at its peak condition.

- Exercise ideas in each State and Territory of Australia you will find the Ministry of Sport and Recreation which supplies information about the types of physical activities that are available in your area.

- Activities may range from badminton lessons to dance classes, canoeing to self defense, tai chi to walking and bushwalking groups. You will discover that there are so many opportunities to meet with others in the community and keep active together.

Ref. Fitness Institute of Research & Education.

BODYBUILDING

Bodybuilding is the act of gain muscle by working out and shaping one's diet to put on more muscle mass. Often bodybuilding is referred to as hard gaining, indicating a regimen tailored for a person without a predisposition towards acquiring muscle mass. Bodybuilding may be done for recreation, for personal betterment or as a competitive sport.

The sport of bodybuilding is judged on the basis of physical appearance and demonstrations of the participants. There is currently a campaign to have bodybuilding adopted as an Olympic sport, but this campaign is met with strong resistance by some sectors. It is commonly argued that bodybuilding is not an actual sport, as the contest itself is non-athletic. When competitive bodybuilders compete, they demonstrate a number of poses intended to accentuate certain muscle groups. This posing is a large part of competitive bodybuilding, and many bodybuilders spent up to half of their training time perfecting their posing routines. Bodybuilding as a sport is not athletic and should not be confused with lifting sports or strongman competitions. The focus on bodybuilding is a specific aesthetic and balance of muscle mass, not feats of strength of agility.

Six pack, eight pack (genetic freaks), washboard, whatever you want to call it, your core is the centerpiece for any muscular physique. It is the eye catcher for the opposite sex. A muscular and well defined core shows both strength and health. Both guys and gals strive to have a strong, toned midsection, but very few of them ever achieve getting one.

In this chapter, we go over the basic anatomy of what makes up the core and list five easy-to-follow workouts to help strengthen your midsection.

Diet and cardiovascular training will have to be in check for you to see your abs. This article will only focus on the training that goes into building and strengthening your mighty core.

Cable Crunches

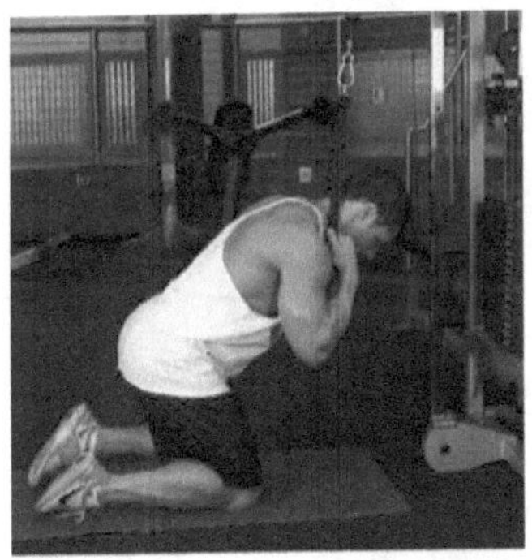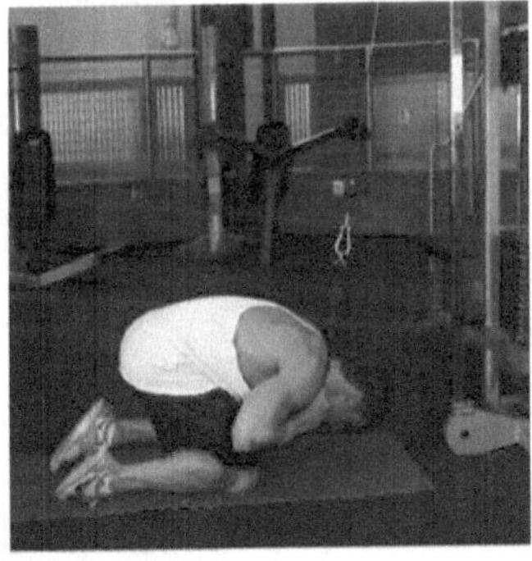

Kneel below a high pulley that contains a rope attachment.

Grasp cable rope attachment and lower the rope until your hands are placed next to your face.

Flex your hips slightly and allow the weight to hyperextend the lower back. This will be your starting position.

With the hips stationary, flex the waist as you contract the abs so that the elbows travel towards the middle of the thighs. Exhale as you perform this portion of the movement and hold the contraction for a second. Slowly return to the starting position as you inhale.

Tip: Make sure that you keep constant tension on the abs throughout the movement. Also, do not choose a weight so heavy that the lower back handles the brunt of the work. Repeat for the recommended amount of repetitions.

Barbell Side Bend

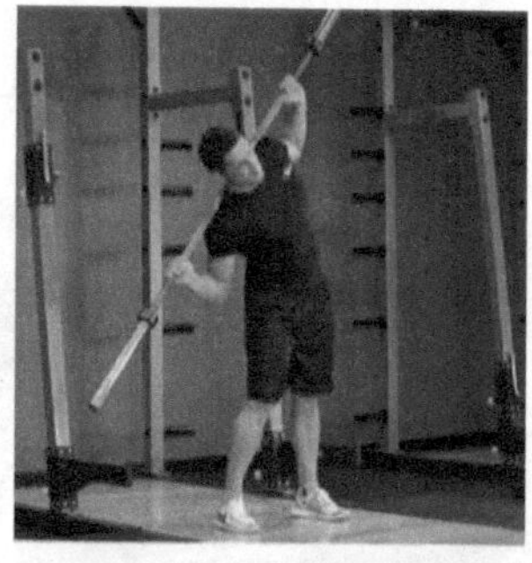

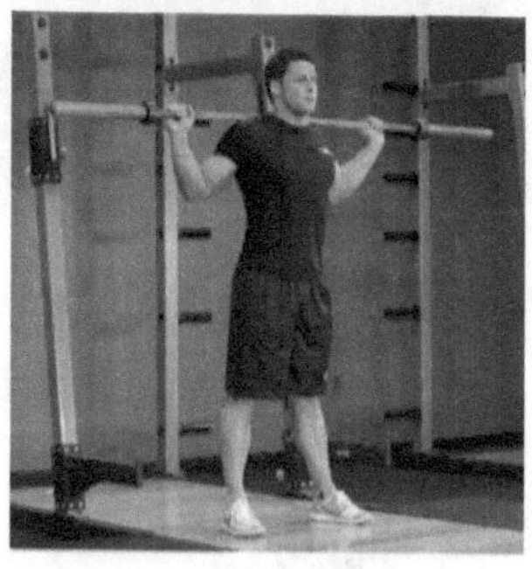

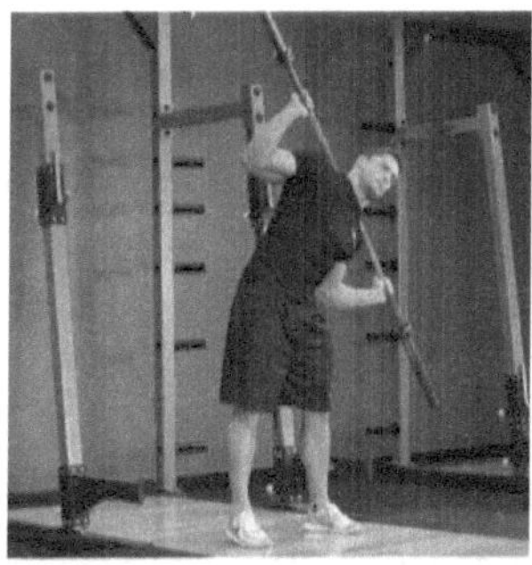

Stand up straight while holding a barbell placed on the back of your shoulders (slightly below the neck). Your feet should be shoulder width apart. This will be your starting position.

While keeping your back straight and your head up, bend only at the waist to the right as far as possible. Breathe in as you bend to the side. Then hold for a second and come back up to the starting position as you exhale.

Tip: Keep the rest of the body stationary. Now repeat the movement but bending to the left side. Hold for a second and come back to the starting position. Repeat for the recommended amount of repetitions.

Caution: Use caution if you have lower back problems, or avoid this exercise altogether.

Reverse Crunches

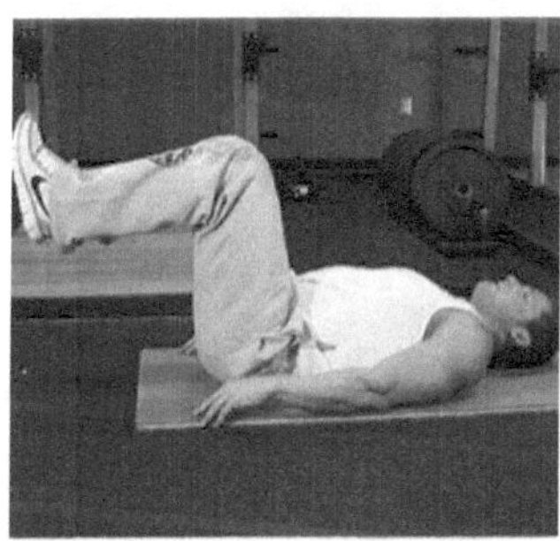

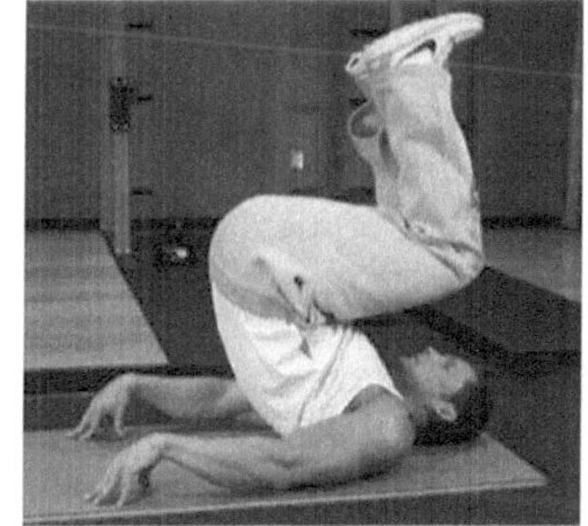

Lie down on the floor with your legs fully extended and arms to the side of your torso with the palms on the floor. Your arms should be stationary for the entire exercise.

Move your legs up so that your thighs are perpendicular to the floor and feet are together and parallel to the floor. This is the starting position.

While inhaling, move your legs towards the torso as you roll your pelvis backwards and you raise your hips off the floor. At the end of this movement your knees will be touching your chest.

Hold the contraction for a second and move your legs back to the starting position while exhaling.

Repeat for the recommended amount of repetitions.

Crunches Overhead

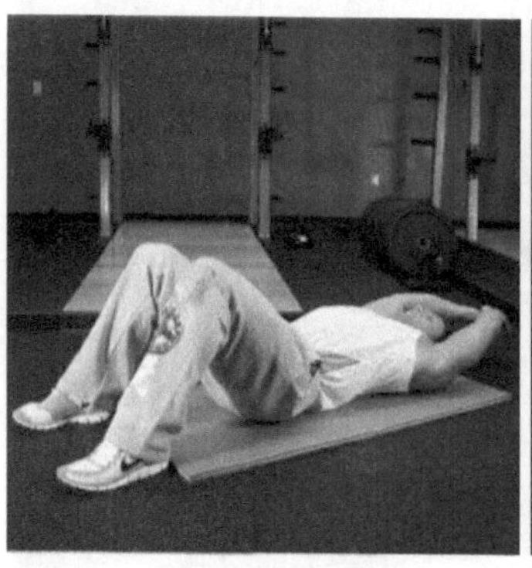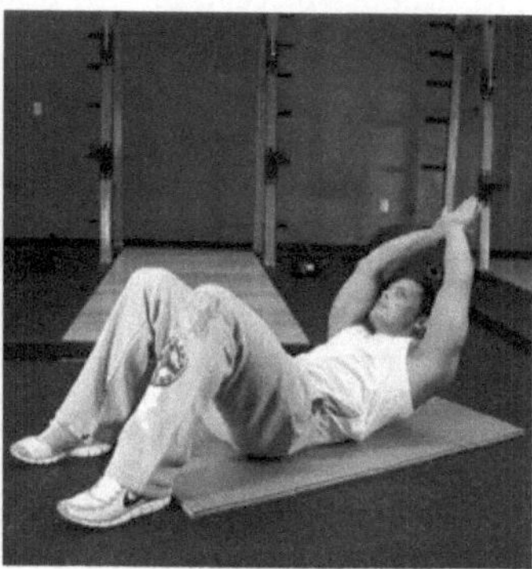

Lie on the floor with your back flat and knees bent with around a 60-degree angle between the hamstrings and the calves.

Keep your feet flat on the floor and stretch your arms overhead with your palms crossed. This will be your starting position.

Curl your upper body forward and bring your shoulder blades just off the floor. At all times, keep your arms aligned with your head, neck and shoulder. Don't move them forward from that position. Exhale as you perform this portion of the movement and hold the contraction for a second.

Slowly lower down to the starting position as you inhale.

Repeat for the recommended amount of repetitions.

Seated Twisting

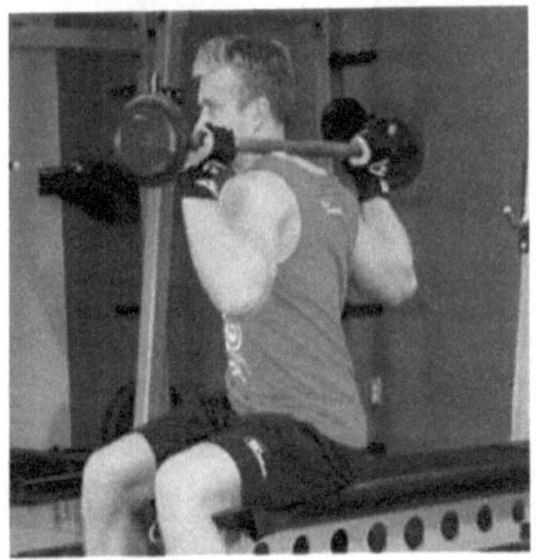 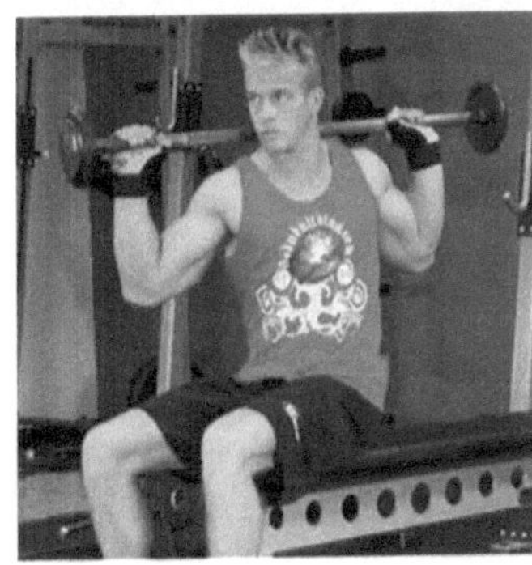

Start out by sitting at the end of a flat bench with a barbell placed on top of your thighs. Your feet should be shoulder width apart from each other.

Grip the bar with your palms facing down and make sure your hands are wider than shoulder width apart from each other. Begin to lift the barbell up over your head until your arms are fully extended.

Now lower the barbell behind your head until it is resting along the base of your neck. This is the starting position.

While keeping your feet and head stationary, move your waist from side to side so that your oblique muscles feel the contraction. Only move from side to side as far as your waist will allow you to go. Stretching or moving too far can cause an injury to occur.

Tip: Use a slow and controlled motion.

Remember to breathe out while twisting your body to the side and in when moving back to the starting position.

Repeat for the recommended amount of repetitions.

Hyper Extension

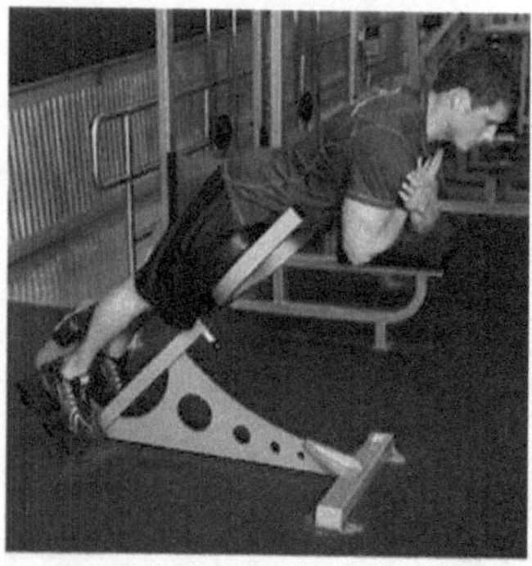
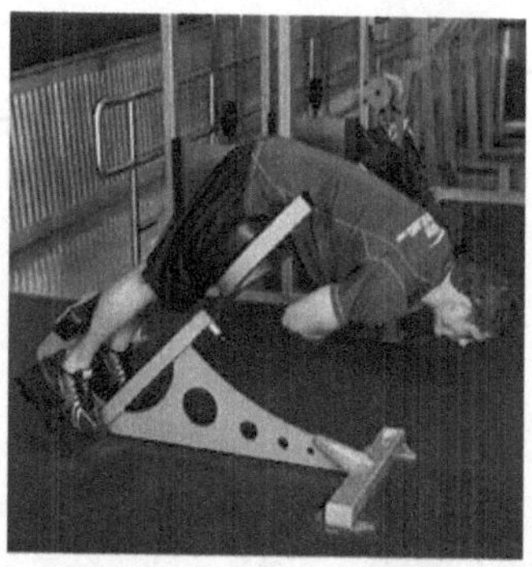

Lie face down on a hyperextension bench, tucking your ankles securely under the footpads.

Adjust the upper pad if possible so your upper thighs lie flat across the wide pad, leaving enough room for you to bend at the waist without any restriction.

With your body straight, cross your arms in front of you (my preference) or behind your head. This will be your starting position.

Tip: You can also hold a weight plate for extra resistance in front of you under your crossed arms.

Start bending forward slowly at the waist as far as you can while keeping your back flat. Inhale as you perform this movement. Keep moving forward until you feel a nice stretch on the hamstrings and you can no longer keep going without a rounding of the back.

Tip: Never round the back as you perform this exercise. Also, some people can go farther than others. The key thing is that you go as far as your body allows you to without rounding the back.

Slowly raise your torso back to the initial position as you inhale.

Tip: Avoid the temptation to arch your back past a straight line. Also, do not swing the torso at any time in order to protect the back from injury.

Repeat for the recommended amount of repetitions.

WEIGHTLIFTING

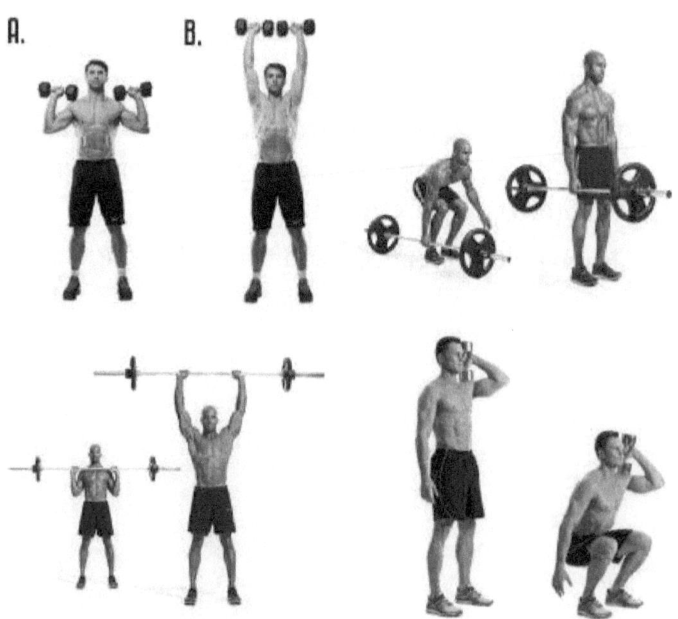

Olympic weightlifting, also called Olympic-style weightlifting, or weightlifting, is an athletic discipline in the modern Olympic programme in which the athlete attempts a maximum-weight single lift of a barbell loaded with weight plates.

The two competition lifts in order are the snatch and the clean and jerk. Each weightlifter receives three attempts in each, and the combined total of the highest two successful lifts determines the overall result within a bodyweight category. Bodyweight categories are different for women and men. A lifter who fails to complete at least one successful snatch and one successful clean and jerk also fails to total, and therefore receives an "incomplete" entry for the competition. The clean and press was once a competition lift, but was discontinued due to difficulties in judging proper form.

In comparison with other strength sports, which test limit strength, Olympic weightlifting tests of human ballistic limits (explosive strength) and are therefore executed faster and with more mobility and a greater range of motion during their execution than other lifts? Properly executed, the snatch and the clean and jerk are both dynamic and explosive while appearing graceful, especially when viewed from a recording at a slower speed.

While there are relatively few competitive Olympic weightlifters, the lifts performed in the Olympics, and in particular their component lifts, are commonly used by elite athletes in other sports to train for both explosive and functional strength.

The sole elements of what is today's modern Olympic weightlifting program the snatch and the clean and jerk. The snatch consists of lifting the barbell from the floor to an overhead position in one fluid motion. It is a very precise lift that can be nullified by a lack of balance of the athlete. The clean and jerk consists of moving the barbell from the floor to overhead in two.

POWER LIFTING

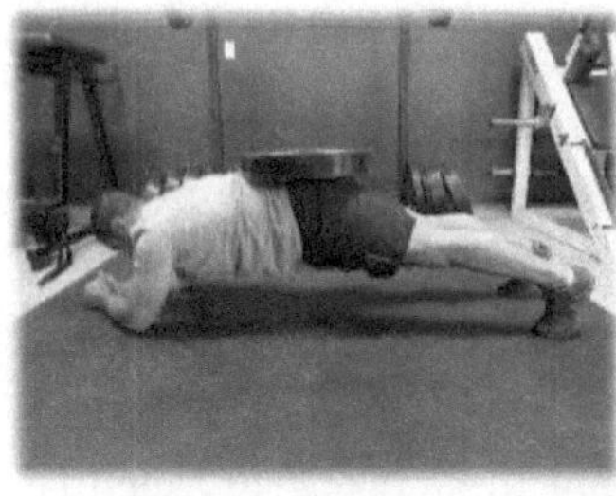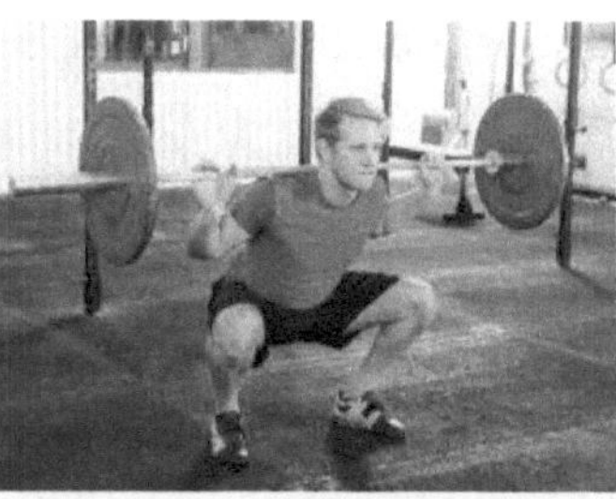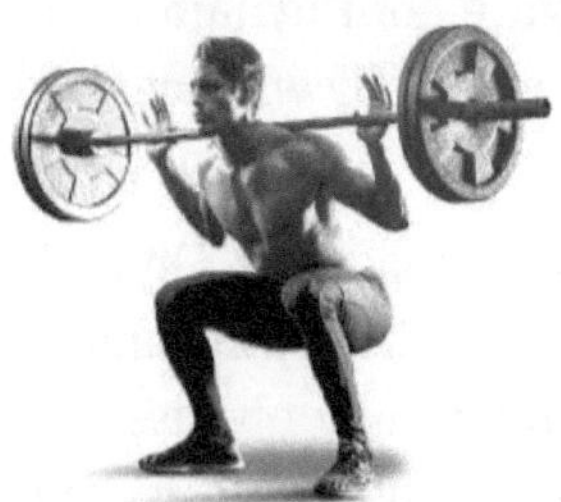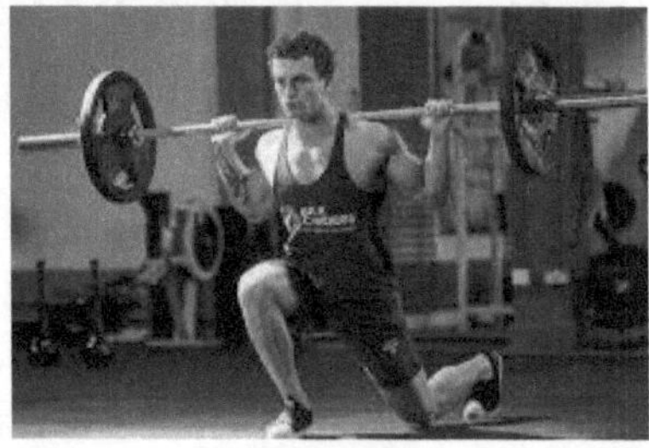

Power lifting is a strength sport that consists of three attempts at maximal weight on three lifts: squat, bench press, and dead lift. As in the sport of Olympic weightlifting, it involves lifting weights in three attempts. Power lifting evolved from a sport known as "odd lifts," which followed the same three-attempt format but used a wider variety of events, akin to strongman competition. Eventually odd lifts became standardized to the current three.

In competition, lifts may be performed equipped or un-equipped (typically referred to as 'raw' lifting or 'classic' in the IPF specifically). Equipment in this context refers to a supportive bench shirt or squat/dead lift suit or briefs. In some federations, knee wraps are permitted in the equipped but not un-equipped division; in others, they may be used in both equipped and un-equipped lifting. Weight belts, knee sleeves, wrist wraps and special footwear may also be used, but are not considered when distinguishing equipped from un-equipped lifting.

Competitions take place across the world but mostly in the United States, Canada, Iceland, Egypt, Sweden, Finland,Russia and Ukraine. Power lifting has been a Paralympics sport since 1984 and, under the IPF, is also a World Games sport. Local, national and international competitions have also been sanctioned by other federations operating independently of the IPF. Effects power lifting

Power lifting has chronic effects with the body of the athlete. Most common effects of the lifts have negative connotations. Most common thoughts about lifting provide skepticism with damage to joints, ligaments and muscles. Also, power lifting is frowned upon by athletic trainers and coaches worldwide due to the belief that will take away from the athletes' functionality "in game." In fact, studies show that power lifting (if trained safely and correctly) creates explosive strengths for athletes to use in powerful short bursts. This type of training, combined with lean muscle weightlifting exercises, can create the best-rounded athletes, and can cause them to build muscular stamina, strength, and explosiveness. A combination of traditional weightlifting with power lifting can create rapid gains for lifters. Normally, lifters plateau rather quickly because of muscular plasticity, but this type of lifting shocks the muscles and allow them to gain exponentially rather than plateau so early. These power lifts (bench, squat, dead lift) increase diaphragm activation as measured by an increase in the Trans diaphragmatic pressure. Studies show that diaphragm thickness is significantly healthier in world class power lifters than those of the control group, or not being exposed to such training. With poor form, training, and lack of lifting maturity, power lifting can be severely dangerous to the body, but with the correct training anyone can achieve healthy, smart, functional, explosive yet lean muscles.

BOOT CAMP

A fitness boot camp is a type of group physical training program conducted by gyms, personal trainers, and former military personnel. These programs are designed to build strength and fitness through a variety of intense group intervals over a one hour period of time. Originally popular in the US, they were brought over to the UK in 1999 and have been growing in popularity ever since.

Boot Camp training often commences with dynamic stretching and running, followed by a wide variety of interval training, including lifting weights/objects, pulling rubber TRX straps, pushups/sit ups, plyometrics, and various types of intense explosive routines. Sessions usually finish with yoga stretching. Many other exercises using weights or body weight, similar to Cross Fit routines, are used to lose body fat, increase cardiovascular efficiency, increase strength, and help people to get into a routine of regular exercise. Many programs offer nutrition advice as well. It is called "boot camp" because it trains groups of people, may be outdoors, and may or may not be similar to military basic training.

The term boot camp is currently used in the fitness industry to describe group fitness classes that promote fat loss, camaraderie, and team effort. They are designed to push people a little bit further than they would normally push themselves in the gym alone. Boot Camps are sometimes organized outdoors in parks using bodyweight exercises like pushups, squats, suspension training and burpees, interspersed with running and competitive games. The idea is that everyone involved works at their own pace as they team up and work towards one goal, either in pairs, small teams of three or four, or even two teams head on.

Boot camps provide social support for those taking part. This provides a different environment for those exercisers who get bored in a gym and so find it hard to develop a habit of exercise. Participants make friends and socialize as they exercise, although how strict the trainers or drill instructors depend on the company running the camp. Members of fitness boot camps are usually tested for fitness on the first day and then retested at the end of the camp, which usually runs for between four and six weeks.Fitness boot camps are often based on the military style of training, although that has started changing over the last few years. An advantage of a boot camp is that the large group dynamic will often help to motivate the participants. A growing trend in fitness boot camps are the indoor locations which prove to be climate proof and provide a better workout environment for the members. Additionally, some camps include extracurricular fitness activities off-site.

There are many other benefits of a fitness boot camp, which includes mental health. It has long been known that regular aerobic exercise can help to reduce high blood pressure, hypertension and combat stress. Part of this is due to the release of endorphins, which act as a mood elevator.

Some Holistic Boot camps provide the mental coaching required sustaining motivation after people leave the camp. Themed fitness boot camps often consist of the use of one particular training implement to the exclusion of others.

Kettle bells are the preferred tool for kettle bell fitness boot camps run by RKC instructors and TRX suspension trainers are the preferred tools for TRX instructors. Boxing themed fitness boot camps often use heavy bags. The use of themes varies widely between fitness boot camps and their instructors according to the preferences between the instructor and the needs and likes of the clientele.

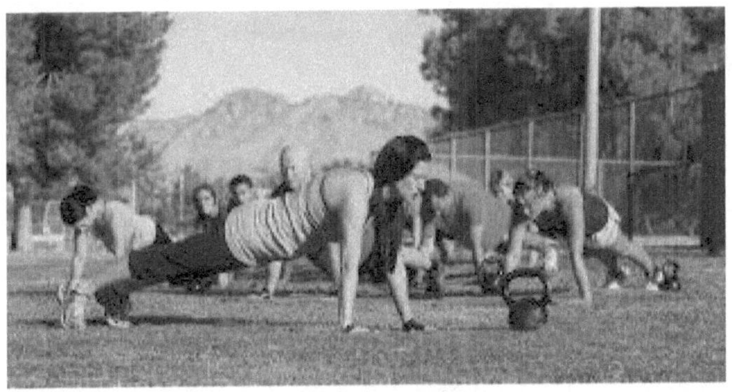

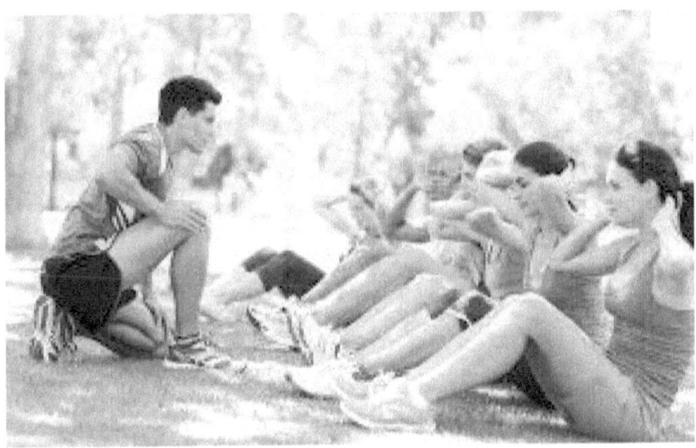

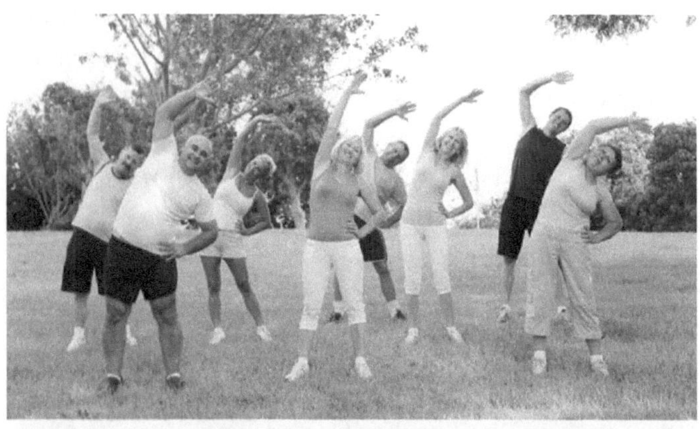

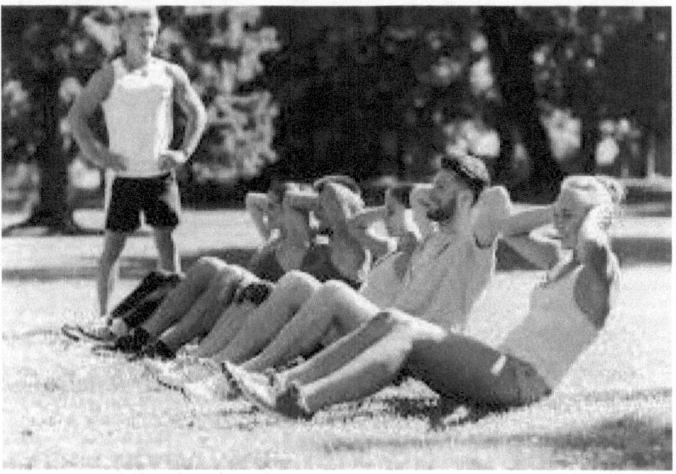

YOGA

Navasana

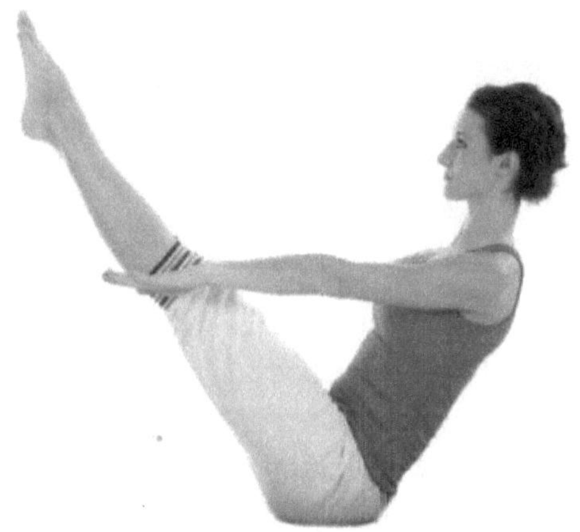

A combination of core strength, hip flexion and mental steadiness, this posture has many different variations so that all levels can practice it. Holding for a minimum of five breaths daily builds powerful core muscles and aligns the spine. A weak core can sometimes create chronic back pain; this posture can be used therapeutically to help alleviate back pain due to weak muscles. Navasana means boat posture in English and it helps to think about hollowing out the pelvis like the inside of a boat to keep the stomach sucked in.

Uttplutih

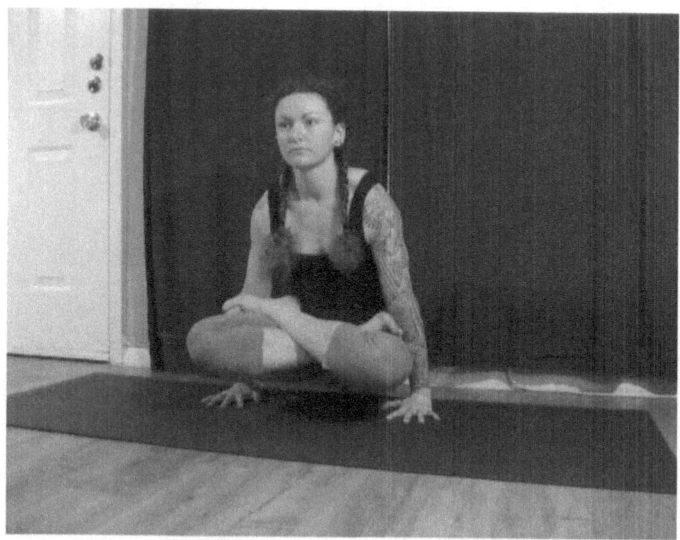

Traditionally the last posture in the rigorous Ashtanga Yoga practice, every muscle in the body engages while pulling into the core of the body. Translated literally as "sprung up," it is best performed with a full lotus position, but can be modified by simply crossing the legs. When the legs are crossed, this is sometimes referred to as Lolasana, but the principle of lifting the entire body off the ground remains the same. The arms, core, thighs and chest are toned. Holding the posture for at least 10 breaths daily builds mental and physical endurance. Practicing this posture directly before taking final rest at the end of your yoga practice helps the muscles relaxed more fully. Combining Navasana with the Lolasana version of the lift up is an integrated part of the Primary Series of Ashtanga Yoga that tests mental limitations as well as physical endurance.

Plank

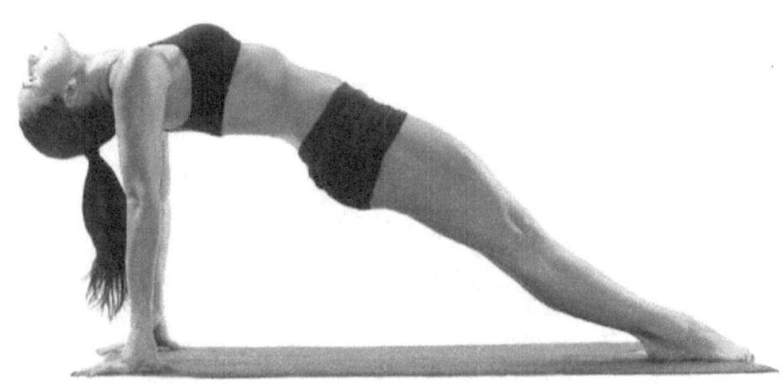

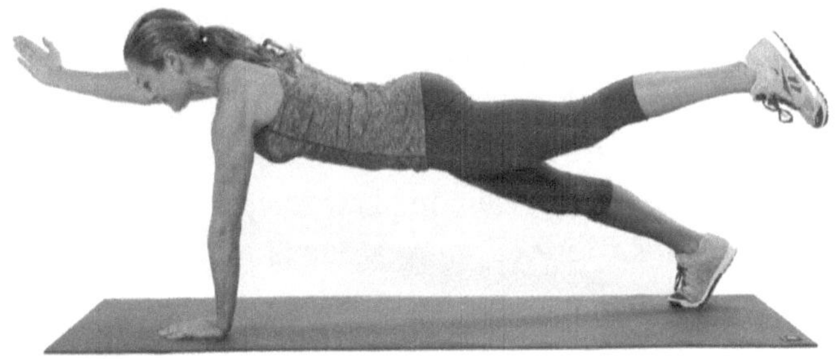

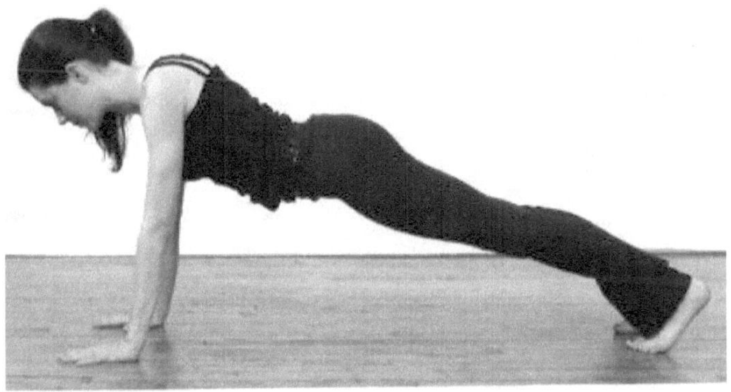

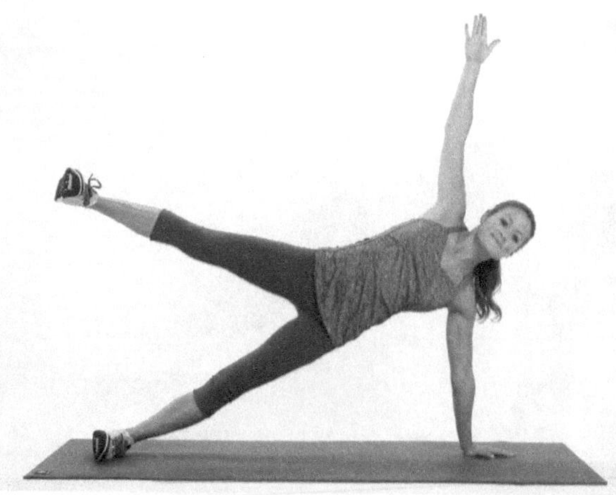

since the arms are straight in these postures almost everyone at all levels of practice can hold the plank position for a solid five breaths. Used as a transition between more challenging postures, the plank holds the basic tools for integration of core strength with upper body power. Directing the mind to remain steady and calm in plank, helps also to calm the nervous system in even more arduous movements, try to hold plank for one minute to really build strength.

Chaturanga Dandasana

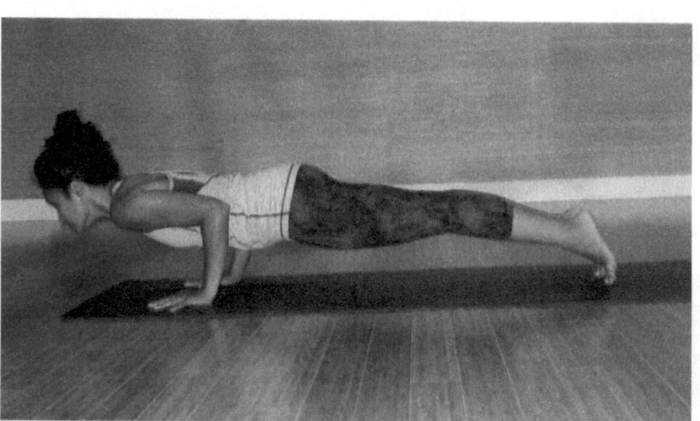

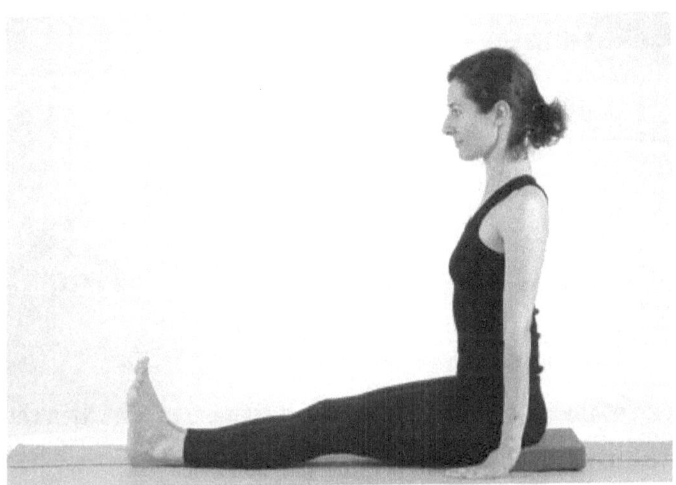

Translated into English as the four-pronged staff posture, this yoga push up position builds healthy shoulder alignment when done properly. Be careful if you do not have good upper body strength because it can be difficult to keep the shoulders in a healthy position. Repetitive movement through Chaturanga Dandasana throughout daily and yoga practice builds inner determination and solidity in strength. Since the elbows are bent rather than straight, a conscious activation of the entire shoulder girdle is necessary in order to prevent injury and build strength. Once you are proficient in both Plank and Chaturanga Dandasana see if you can combine both movements to go up and down, initiating the push up from the core of the body rather than just the arms. In this posture, position of shoulders is important for building solid strength.

Bakasana

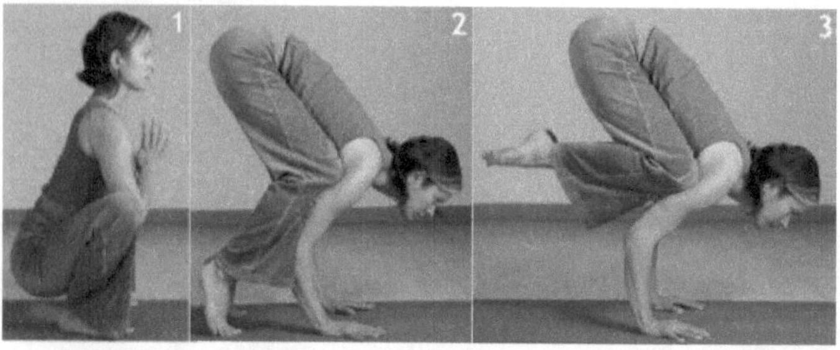

one of the most fundamental of all arm balances, when the student truly masters this posture, most other arm balances is possible. In the ideal position the knees rest in the hollows of the armpits. It is important to engage the shoulder girdle while flexing the spine and firming the pelvic floor to integrate the deep work of Bakasana. Used as a transition repeatedly from other more challenging arm balances, it is crucial to be fully established in regular practice of Bakasana in order to develop strength in yoga. However, if you rush into the posture without proper development of the core, it may put strain of the wrists so proceed with caution. If you are proficient in the posture you can try jumping directly back into Chaturanga Dandasana, jumping into the posture from Downward Facing Dog or entering and exiting Bakasana from Handstand.

Astavakrasana

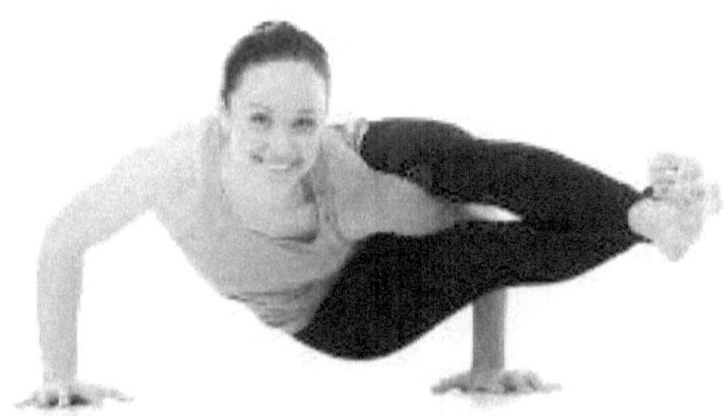

Translated as eight angle posture, this asymmetrical arm balance will build symmetrical strength in your shoulders over time. By practicing both sides equally your shoulders and core will learn to support the weight of the body. Traditionally practiced in the arm balance sequence of the Third Series of Ashtanga Yoga, do not underestimate the level of difficulty needed in order to find stability in and out of the posture.

Handstand

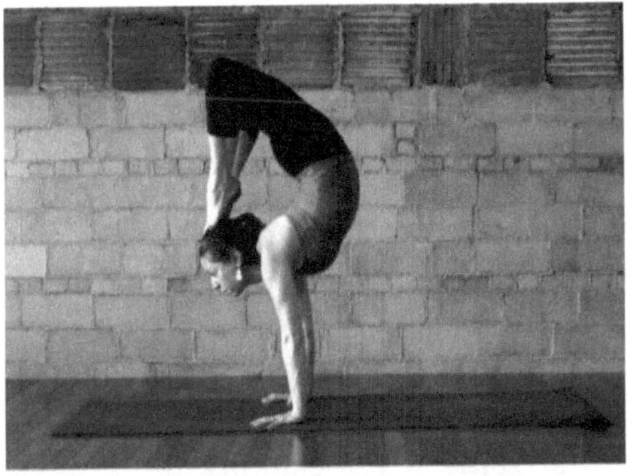

One of the greatest tests of all inversions, balancing fully on your hands requires strength of mind and body. If your mind wavers while you attempt a handstand you will most certainly fall. Strong shoulders and core are needed for a stable handstand mastery Once the handstand is mastered it can be used to further develop strength through transitions into and out of other arm balances such as Bakasana.

Headstand

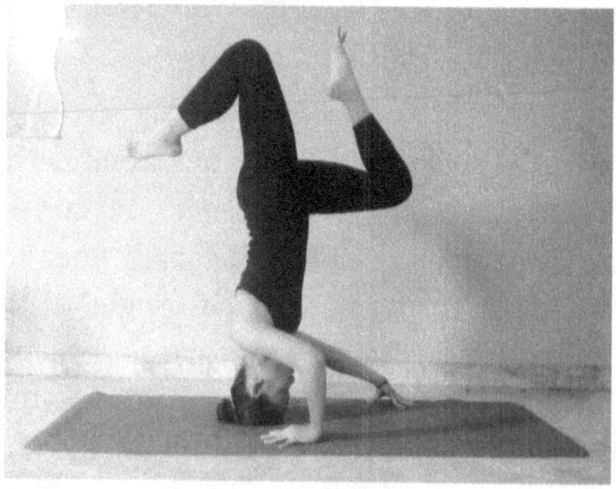

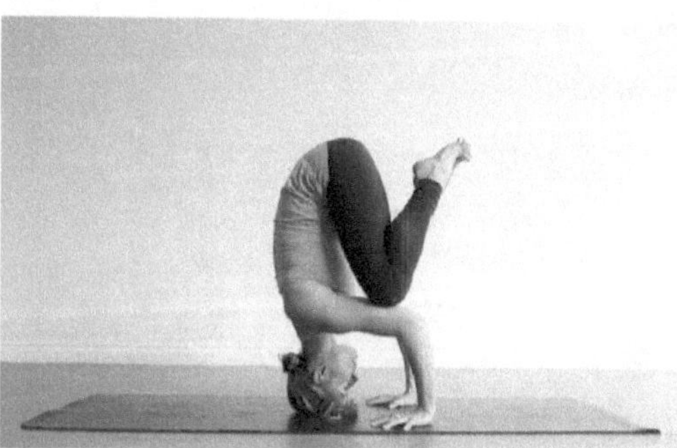

The most basic and perhaps healing inversion, headstand, known in Sanskrit as Sirsasana, tests the alignment of the shoulders and spine while calming the nervous system.

Traditionally done as a Closing Posture when the mind is meant to be moving more towards a meditative state, headstand can be held for long periods of time, sometimes as long as twenty minutes. However, beginners are recommended to start off with only 10 breaths and increase slowly as strength and alignment improve. Long periods of time spent in Sirsasana create mental stability and focus.

Pinchamayurasana

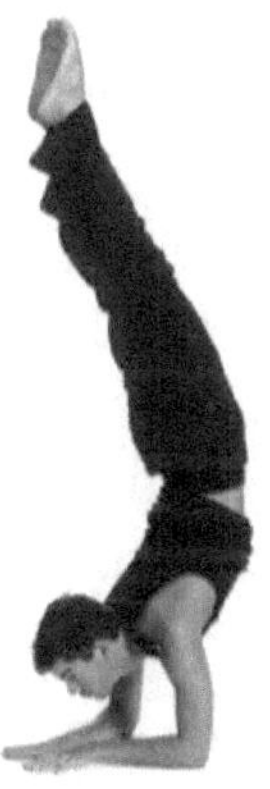

Increasing the activation and strength required for headstand, Pinchamayurasana is a forearm balance that demands a conscious activation of the shoulder girdle and the core of the body. If your shoulder collapses or pinches forward this is not a safe posture. If your core is too weak and your spine extends into a backbend the alignment of your spine will be compromised. Regular practice helps the students and individual learn howto press through their foundation, align the spine and strengthen the shoulders. Finding the balance point in Pinchamayurasana pose helps to build mental and emotional balance as well.

Vishwamitrasana

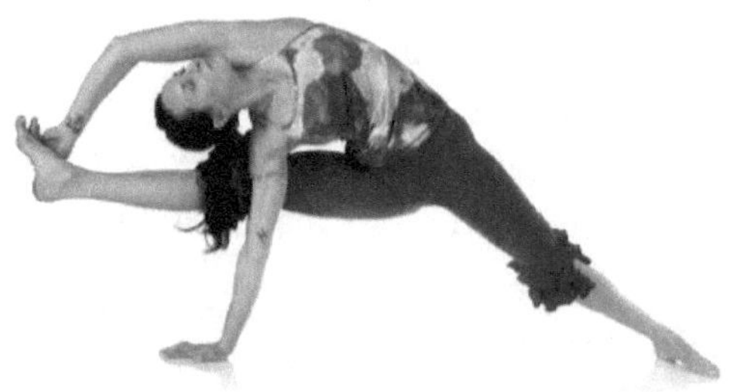

Named after the sage Vishwamitra, this posture is the first of the challenging third series of Ashtanga Yoga. It is sometimes called Vashistasana is other styles of yoga, but it is nonetheless the same posture. Built on a one arm side plank this posture tests alignment in the shoulders and of core of the body, Regular practice will even out asymmetries in strength and build steadiness of mind.

Abdominal Strengthening, when instructed place your hands to your thighs.

Inhale then as you exhale lifts your pelvic floor and your stomach muscles and slowly curls up lifting your shoulders from your mat.

As you inhale slowly, uncurl and release your pelvic floor muscles returning to your starting position.

Continue as instructed. When instructed, place your fingertips to your temples. Inhale then as you exhale lift your pelvic floor and your stomach muscles and slowly curl up lifting your shoulders from your mat.

As you inhale slowly un-curl and release your pelvic floor muscles returning to your starting position. Continue as instructed. When instructed, exhale as you do so lift your pelvic floor and your stomach muscles and slowly curl up directing your right shoulder to towards your left knee.

Continue on each side as instructed.

AEROBICS

Aerobic Exercise

Imagine that you're exercising. You're working up a sweat, you're breathing hard, your heart is thumping, blood is coursing through your vessels to deliver oxygen to the muscles to keep you moving, and you sustain the activity for more than just a few minutes. That's aerobic exercise also known as cardio in gym ling, Any activity that you can sustain for more than just a few minutes that's mean your heart, lungs, and muscles work overtime. In this chapter, I have discussed the mechanisms of aerobic exercise: oxygen transport and consumption, the role of the heart and the muscles, the proven benefits of aerobic exercise, how much you need to do to reap the benefits, and more.

Beginning

It all starts with breathing. The average healthy adult inhales and exhales about 7 to 8 liters of air per minute. Once you fill your lungs, the oxygen in the air (air contains approximately 20% oxygen) is filtered through small branches of tubes (called bronchioles) until it reaches the alveoli. The alveoli are microscopic sacs where oxygen diffuses (enters) into the blood. From there, it's a beeline direct to the heart.

The heart has four chambers that fill with blood and pump blood (two atria and two ventricles) and some very active coronary arteries. Because of all this action, the heart needs a fresh supply of oxygen, and the lungs provide it. Once the heart uses what it needs, it pumps the blood, the oxygen, and other nutrients out through the large left ventricle and through the circulatory system to all the organs, muscles, and tissues that need it.

Your heart beats approximately 60–80 times per minute at rest, 100,000 times a day, more than 30 million times per year, and about 2.5 billion times in a 70-year lifetime! Every beat of your heart sends a volume of blood (called stroke volume), along with oxygen and many other life-sustaining nutrients, circulating through your body. The average healthy adult heart pumps about 5 liters of blood per minute.

Oxygen Consumption

All that oxygen being pumped by the blood is important. You may be familiar with the term "oxygen consumption." In science, its labeled Vo_2, or volume of oxygen consumed. It's the amount of oxygen the muscles extract, or consume from the blood, and it's expressed as ml/kg/minute (milliliters per kilogram of body weight). Muscles are like engines that run on fuel (just like an automobile that runs on fuel); only our muscles use fat and carbohydrates instead of gasoline. Oxygen is a key player because, once inside the muscle, it's used to burn fat and carbohydrate for fuel to keep our engines running. The more efficient our muscles are at consuming oxygen, the more fuel we can burn, the more fit we are, and the longer we can exercise.

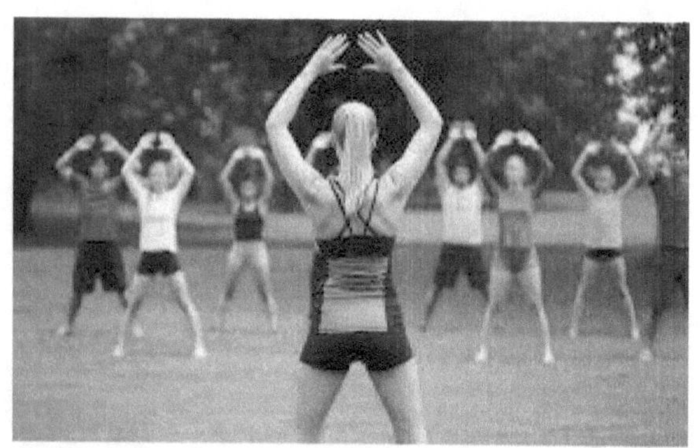

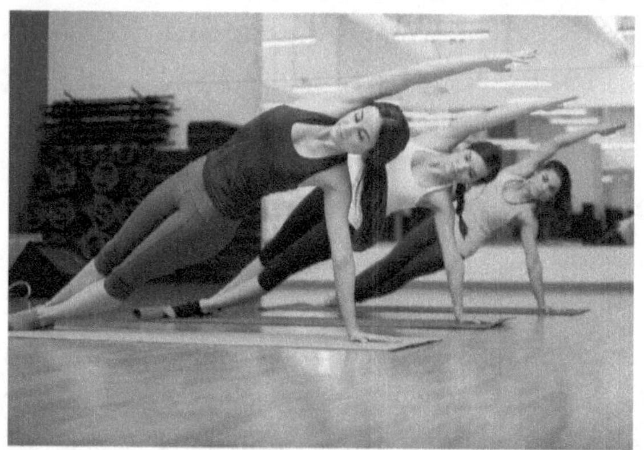

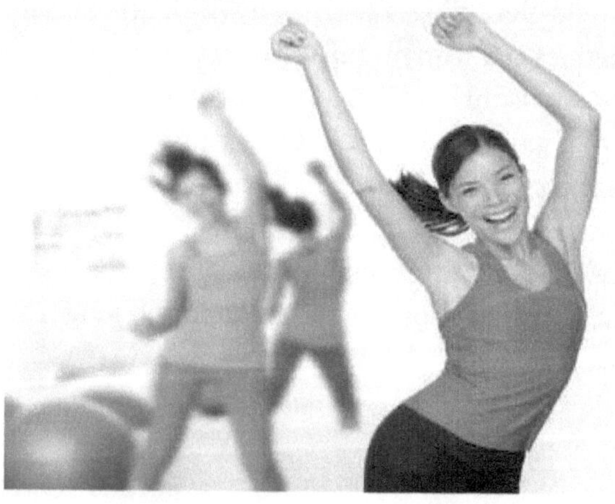

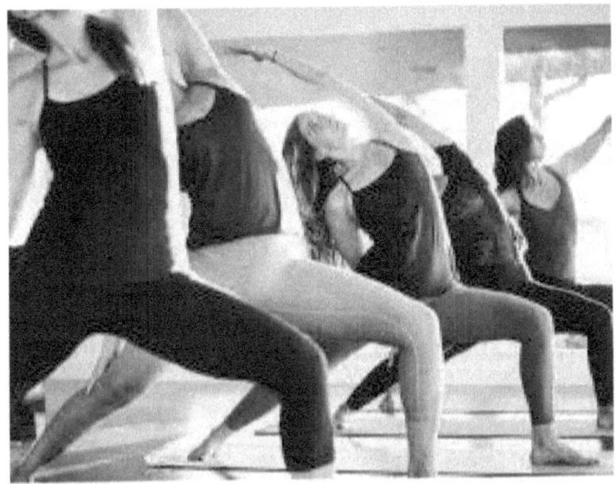

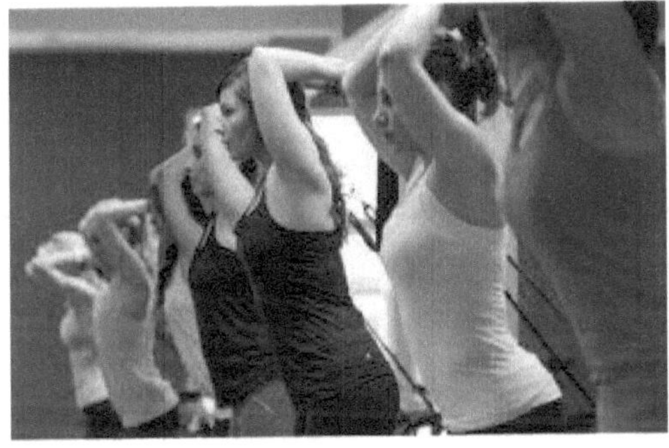

MAT PILATES

Joseph Pilates believed the purpose of his work was to help people to function better in every aspect of their daily life not just when they were exercising. The Pilates method focuses on practicing with awareness and attention to proper form in order to train the body to move with strength, grace and efficiency. Whether you are a professional athlete, a dancer, a computer programmer or a house wife, Pilates exercises are truly "movement for life."

The Pilates method of exercise as Joe called; it was way ahead of its time. Joe focused on complex, functional movement and the essential use of the core at least sixty years before "functional fitness" and "core stabilization" became the foundation of rehabilitation, athletic training and physical fitness programs around the world. The Pilates movement principles are the heart of the method and are used in every exercise both on the mat and on the equipment. The scientific basis behind each principle is included along with exercises to illustrate each principle in action. As you go through this section, practice each exercise several times until you get a good idea of what you are trying to accomplish.

Knee Planks

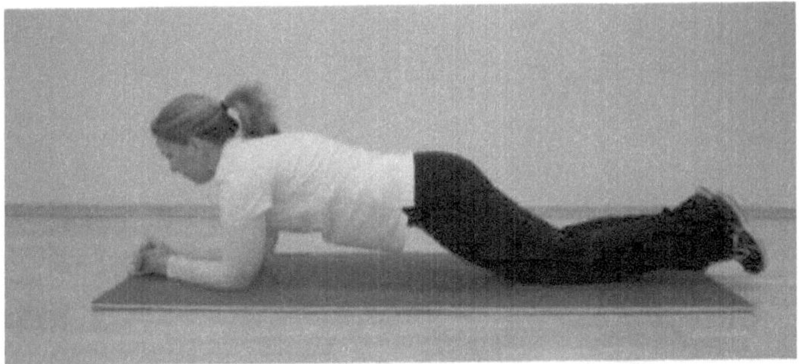

Begin by lying on stomach, elbows bent, and weight on forearms. Lift body up so that weight is on elbows and knees. Keep back as straight as possible contracting the belly into the spine. Do not let hips drop or rise. Remember to breath. Hold for 30 seconds and work up to 1–2 minutes. Repeat for 1–3 sets.

Knee Side Planks

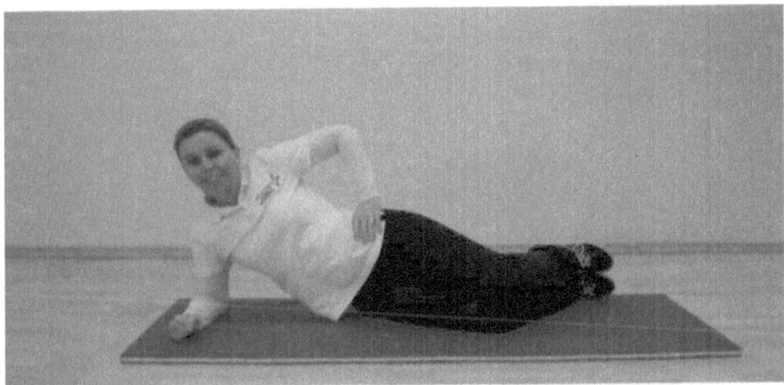

Begin by lying on side with arm bent and resting weight on the elbow. Knees should be bent as well. Lift the body up so that weight is on knee and elbow. Keep body as straight as possible. Hold for 30 seconds and work up to 1–2 minutes. Repeat on each side for 1–3 sets.

Birddog

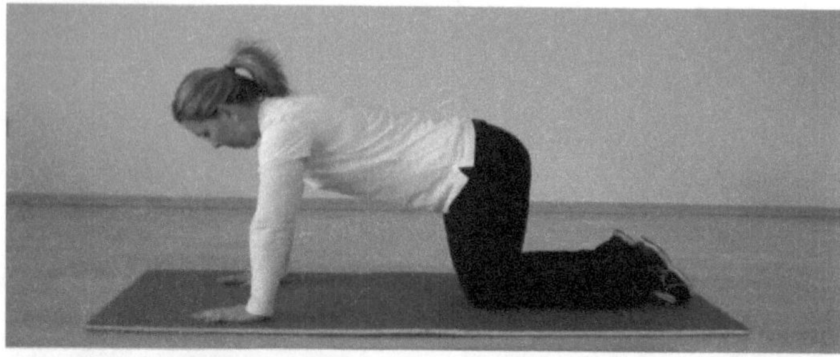

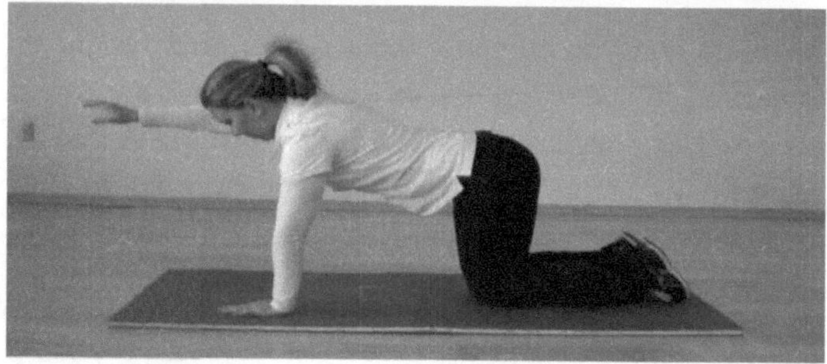

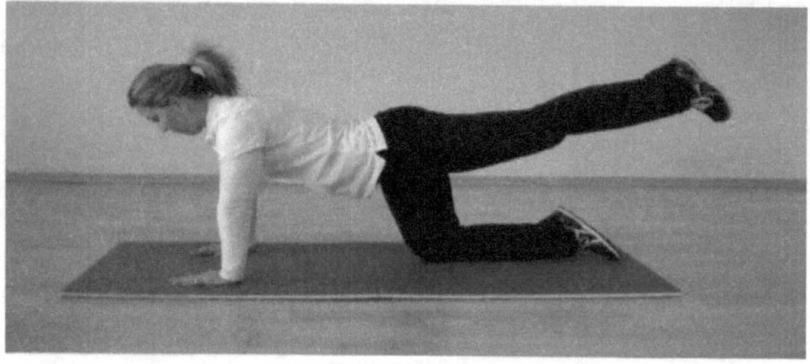

Begin on all fours with hands under shoulders and knees under hips. Keep back straight and head in line with the spine. Extend one arm and hold for 5 seconds. Return to start. Extend the opposite leg and hold for 5 seconds. Return to start. Make sure arm and leg are in level with back. Perform 10 repetitions for each leg/arm combination for 1–3 sets.

Planks

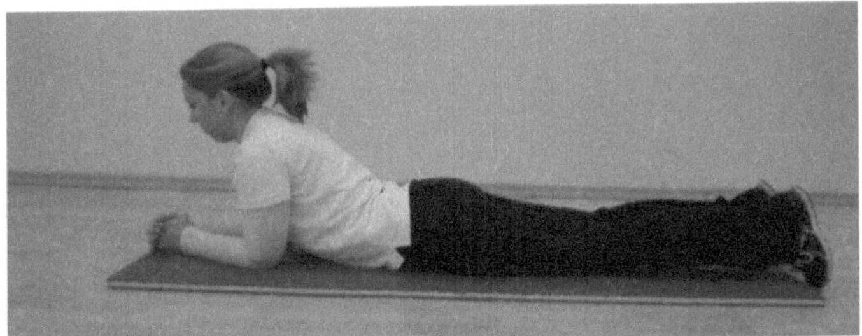

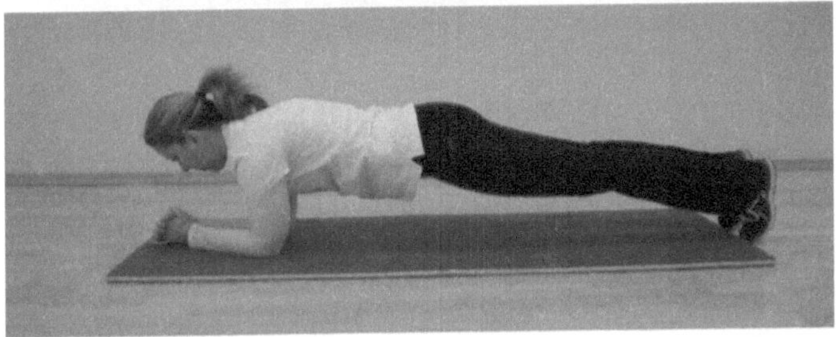

Begin by lying on stomach, elbows bent, and weight on forearms. Lift body up so that weight in on elbows and toes. Keep back as straight as possible keeping the belly tucked in. Do not let hips drop or rise. Remember to breath. Hold for 30 seconds and work up to 1–2 minutes. Repeat for 1–3 sets.

Side Planks

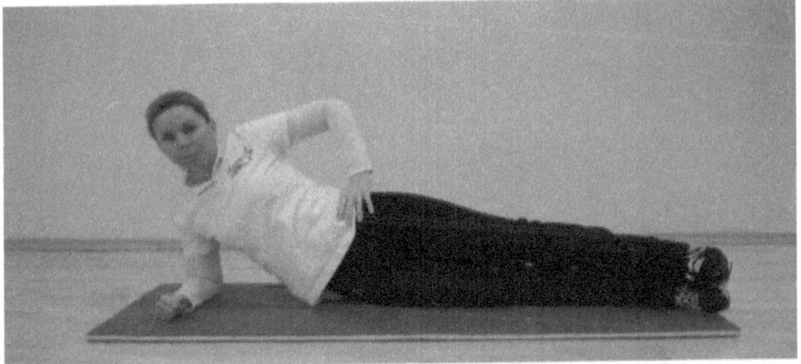

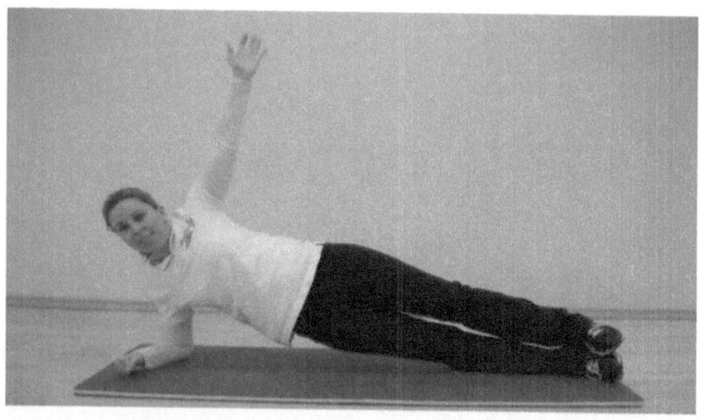

Begin by lying on side with arm bent and resting weight on the elbow. Legs are straight with weight on the outside of the foot in contact with the floor. Lift the body up so that weight is on foot and elbow. Bring your top arm straight up for added difficulty. Keep body as straight as possible. Hold for 30 seconds and work up to 1–2 minutes. Re-peat on each side for 1–3 sets.

Advanced Birddog

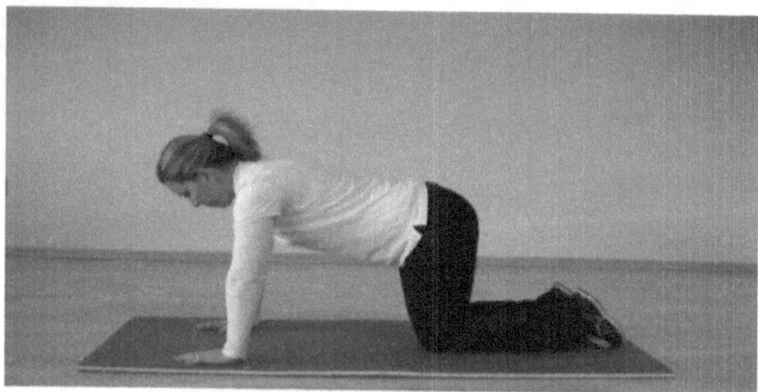

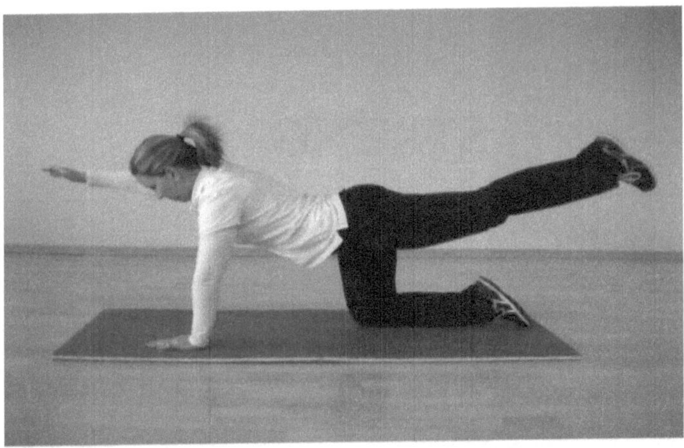

Begin on all fours with hands under shoulders and knees under hips. Without arching back and keeping head in line with spine, extend right arm and left leg up. Make sure arm and leg are level with the back. Balance for 5 seconds before returning to starting position. Perform 10 repetitions for each arm/leg combination for 1–3 sets.

STRENGTH

Crunches

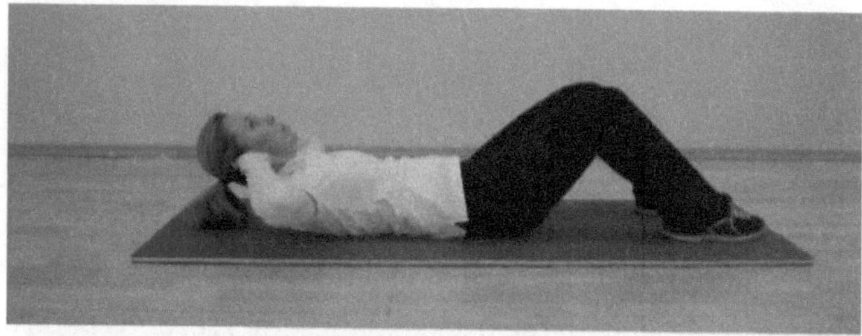

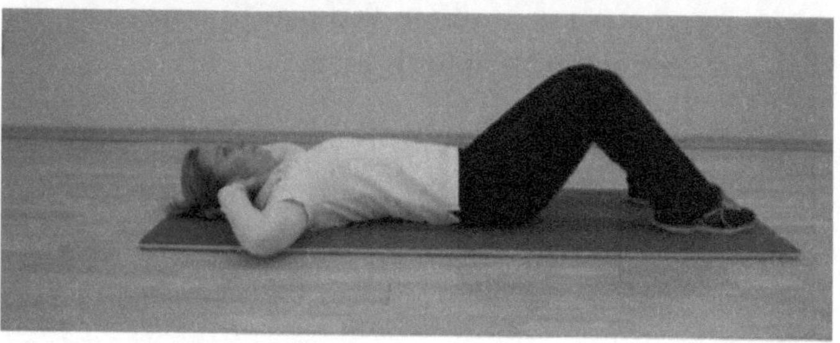

Begin by lying on back with knees bent and hands clasped behind head. Elbows should be out wide. Take a deep breath in and on the exhale lift your shoulders off the floor about 6–12 inches, making sure to not to strain neck by looking up and not tucking chin down. Hold for 1–2 seconds and then return to starting position, Perform 10–20 repetitions for 1–3 sets.

Tips: While perform performing core exercises, breathing is key, Breath out on the contraction

Crunches with Twist

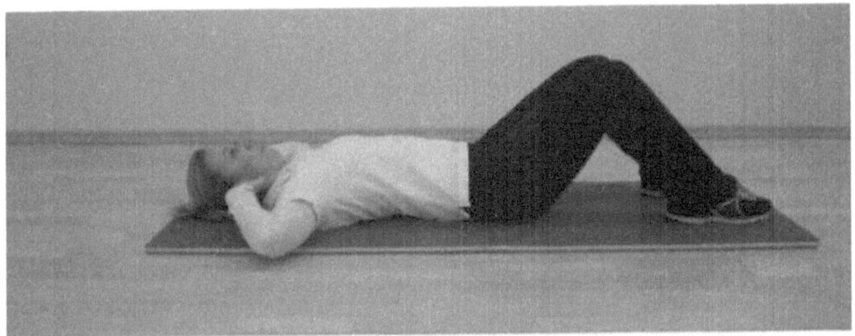

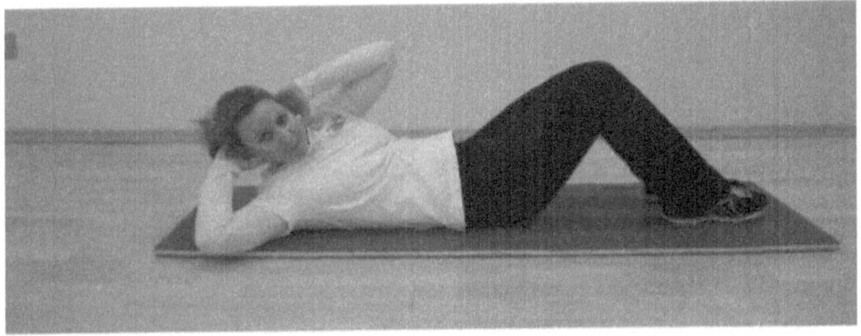

Begin in same position as a crunch. Instead of going straight up, twist to the right then return to starting position. On the next repetition twist to the left and then return to starting position. Perform 10–20 repetitions for 1–3 sets.

Leg Lifts

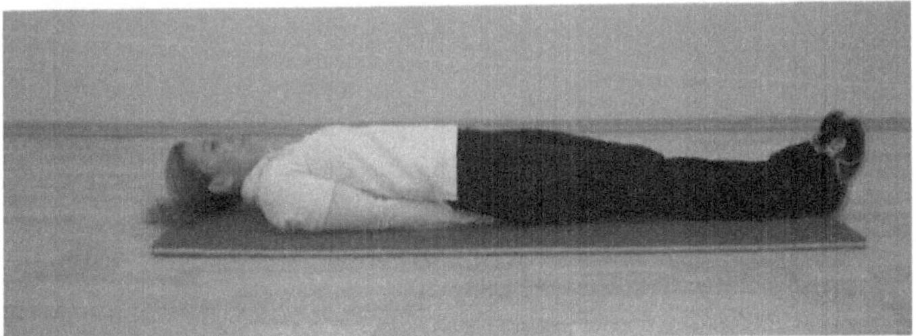

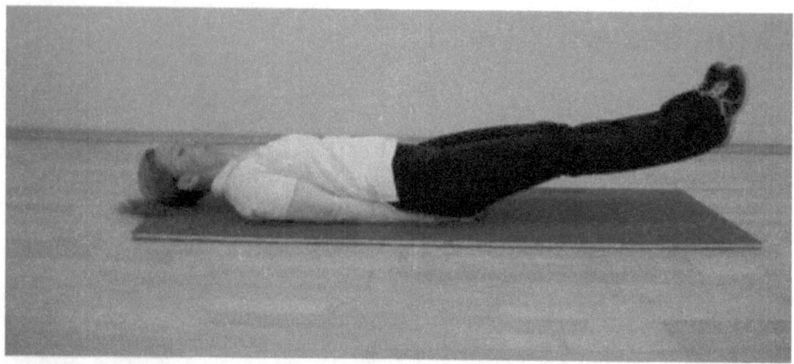

Begin by lying on back with legs flat. Slide hands under rear for satiability and lower back support. Slowly lift legs off the ground about 12 inches and bring back to starting position. If this is difficult, start with one leg at a time until strong enough to lift both or bend the knees slightly. Perform 10–20 repetitions for 1–3 sets.

Reverse Crunch

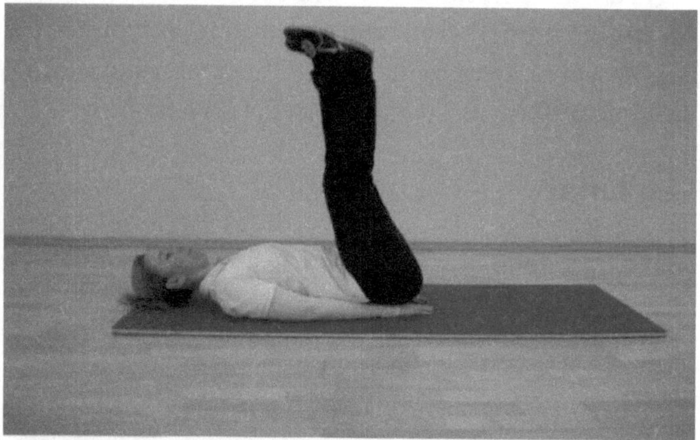

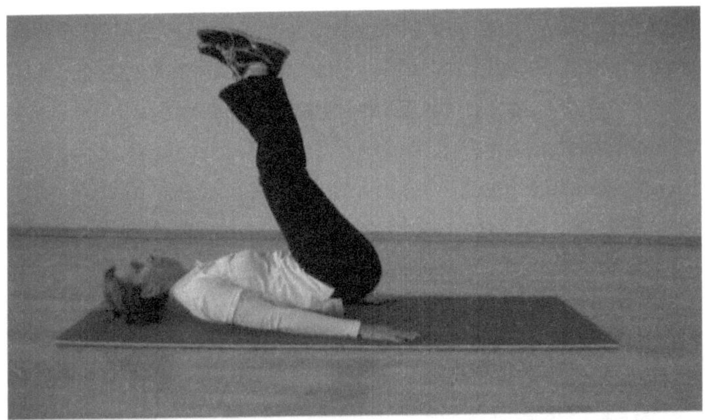

Begin by lying on back with both feet in the air. Lift your pelvis off the floor and return for one repetition. Hands should be flat on the ground at sides for stability. Perform 10–20 repetitions for 1–3 sets.

Classic Wood Chop

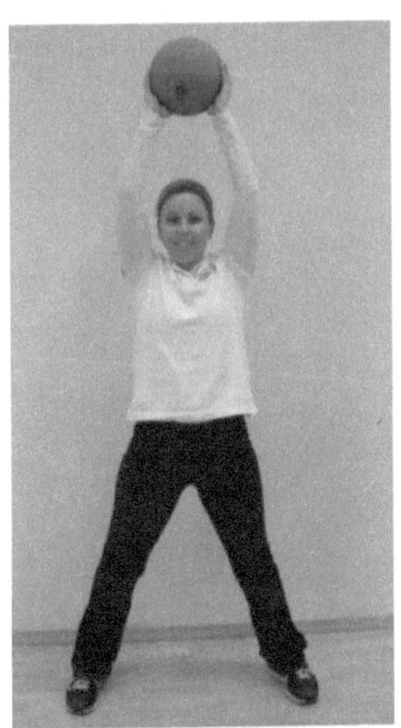

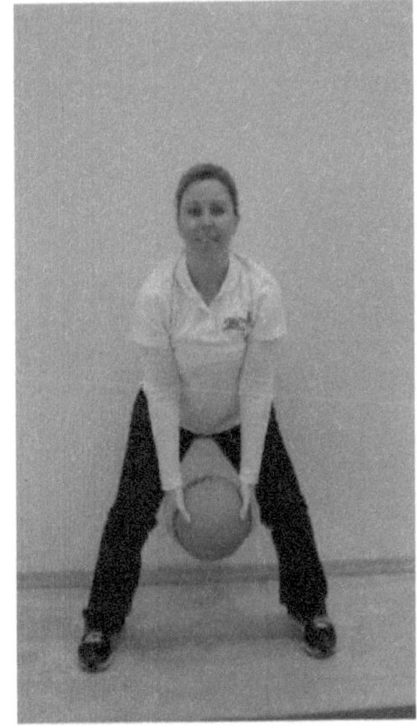

Begin by standing while holding a medicine ball (4–6 lbs). Legs should be slightly wider than shoulders. Raise the ball above head to start. Bend the knees and move hips back when lowering the ball. Arms should stay straight as the ball lowers to knee level. Make sure to keep knees in line with toes and not in front of them. Return to starting position and repeat for 10 repetitions for 1–3 sets.

Crunches with Medicine Ball

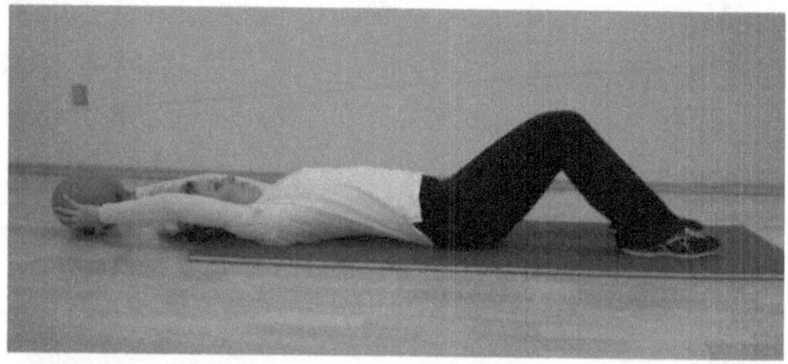

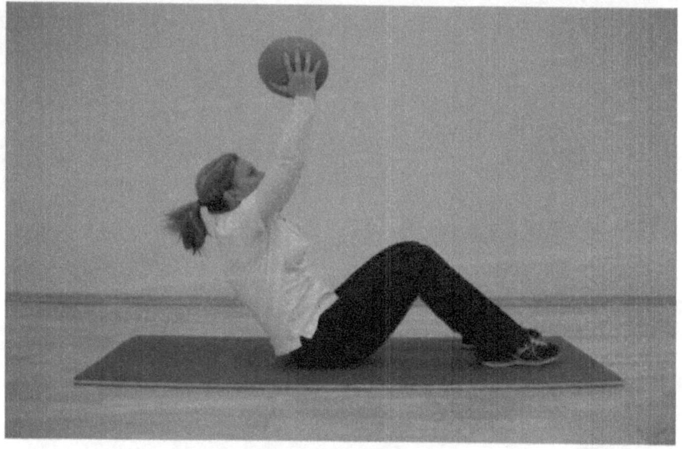

Begin by lying on back with knees bent. Hold the medicine ball with arms straight behind head on the floor. Take a deep breath in and on the exhale lift your torso off the floor about 6–12 inches, making sure not to strain neck by looking up and not tucking chin. Bring arms straight up with ball until back is straight. Hold for 1–2 seconds and return to starting position. Perform 10–20 repetitions for 1–3 sets.

Twist with Medicine Ball

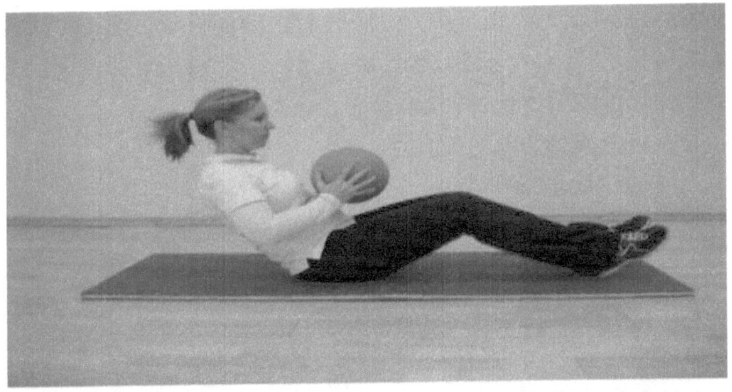

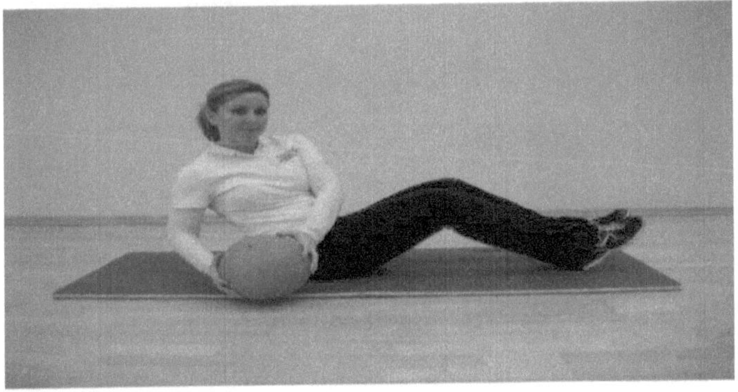

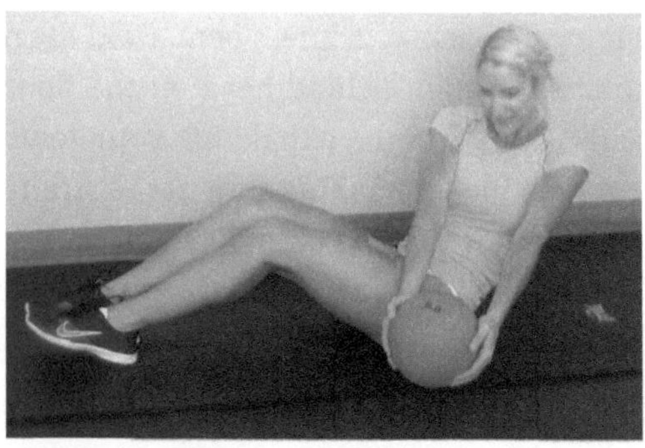

Start in the up position with back off the ground (feet off the ground for even more advanced movement). Twist to the right and left touching the medicine ball to the ground on each side. This exercise can be done at a fast or slow pace. Perform 10–20 repetitions for 1–3 sets.

Core Ball Transfer

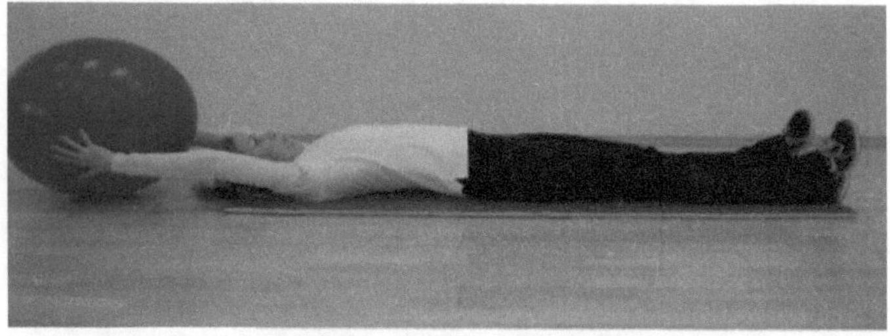

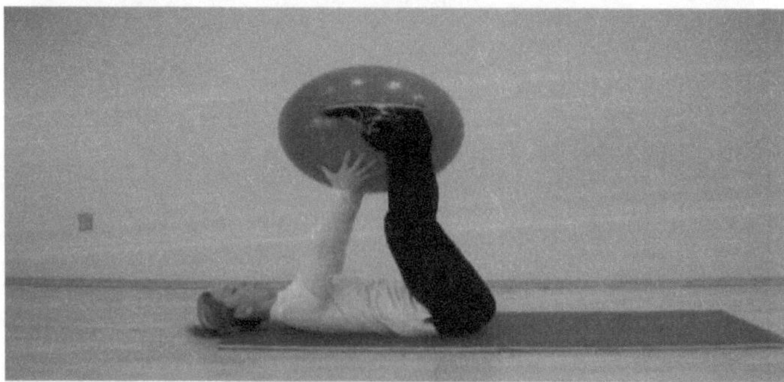

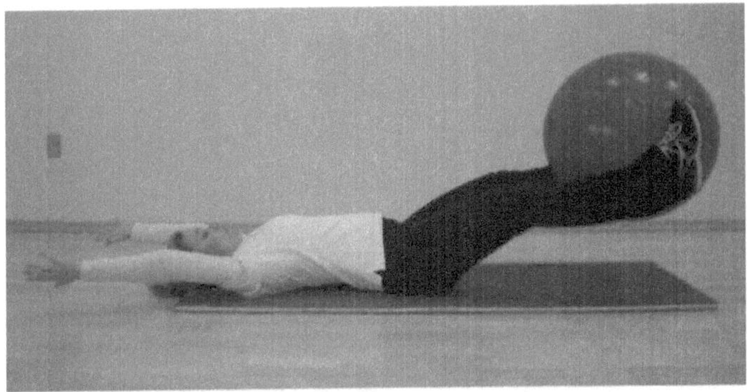

Start on back while holding a core ball above the head. Bring arms and legs up to transfer the ball from your hands to your knees/feet. Return to starting position and repeat, this time transferring from the knees/feet back to the arms. Perform 8–10 repetitions for 1–3 sets.

Knee Tucks with Core Ball

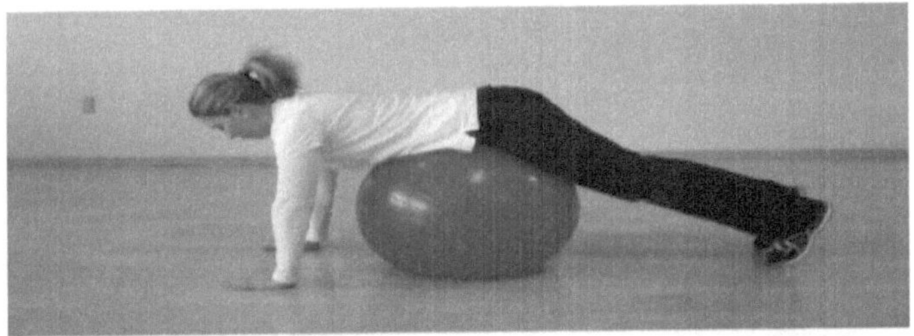

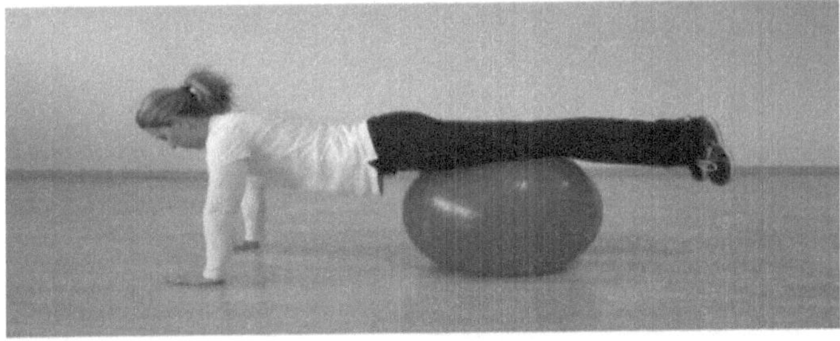

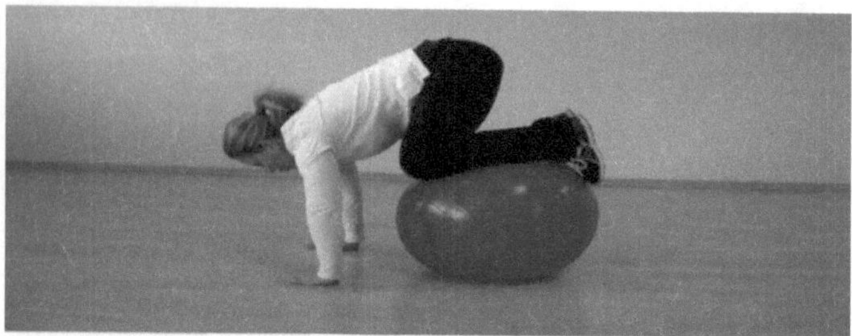

Begin on all fours with ball under torso. Slowly walk hands forward until feet come off floor and thighs are on ball with shoulders in a straight line with hands in the plank position. Exhale and slowly bend knees toward chest as ball rolls closer to arms in a tucked position. The hips will move toward ceiling. The knees should be in line with the hips in the tuck position. Inhale and straighten legs back into starting plank position. Perform 8–10 repetitions for 1–3 sets.

Oblique Wood Chops

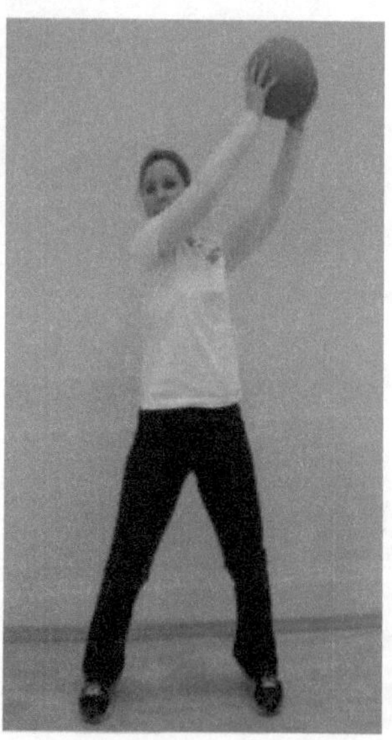

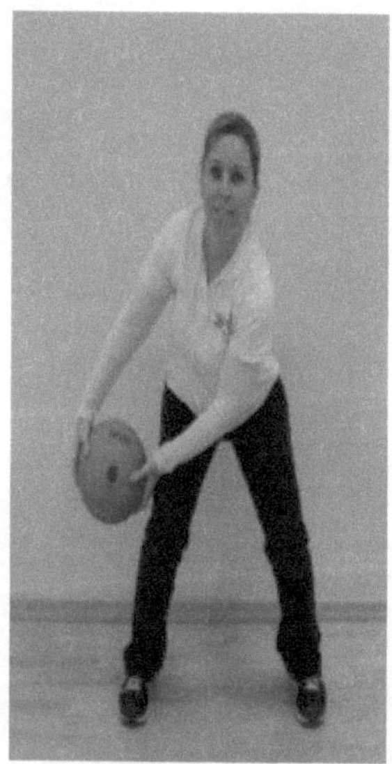

Begin by standing and holding a medicine ball (4–6 lbs). Legs should be slightly wider than shoulders. Raise the ball above head to either the left or right side. Bend the knees as the ball lowers to the outside of the opposite knee. Arms should stay straight as the ball lowers to knee level. Return to starting position and repeat on each side for 10 repetitions for 1–3 sets.

TRX

Whether your fitness aim is to increase your balance and flexibility, while your core into a six pack to be proud of, or lose some serious pounds, all you need is some moveable TRX swag and your own body weight to do it. The most basic TRX equipment is an adjustable cord with two handles, and a pole, tree, or alternative anchor to enfold it around.

Tip: Don't let the TRX straps rest or rub against your arms or legs during the exercise.

TRX Suspended Plank with Abduction

Setup: Adjust the TRX so the lowest point of the foot cradles is 8 to 12 inches from the ground.

Start position: Place your toes in the foot cradles and assume a plank position with your hands or Forearms on the floor, your feet directly beneath the anchor point, and your legs together, the Separate your legs as wide as possible without compromising your body alignment. Pause with your legs at the widest point. Repeat for 30 seconds.

Tip: Make the exercise harder by walking your hands farther away from the anchor point.

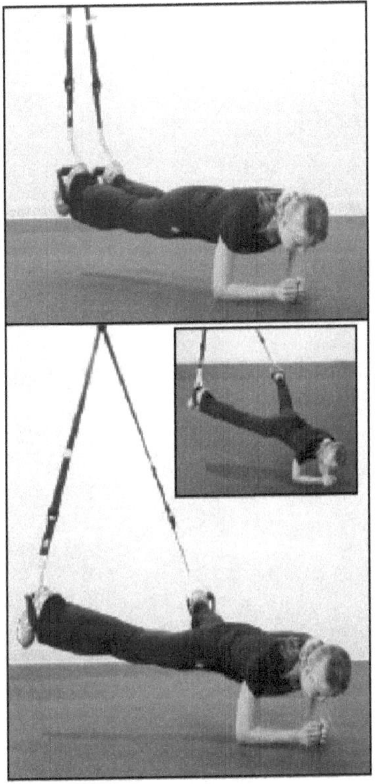

TRX Hip Press

Setup: Adjust the TRX so the lowest point of the foot cradles is 8 to 12 inches from the ground.

Start position: Place your heels inside the footcradles and position your feet directly under the anchor point.

Lie face up on the floor with your arms at your sides, palms flat on the floor.

Press down with your heels, using your core and gluts to lift your hips so your body forms a straight line from shoulders to heels.

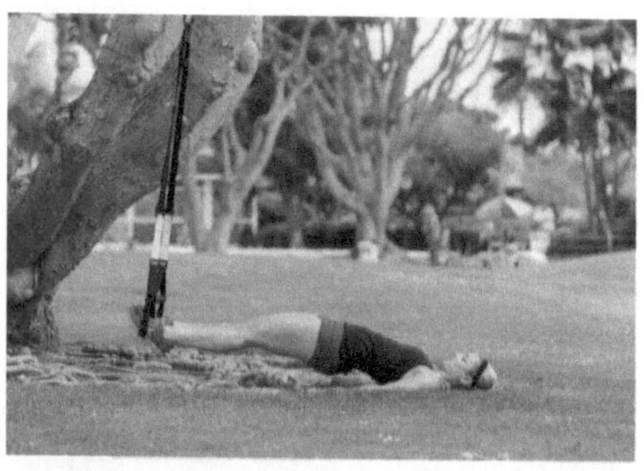

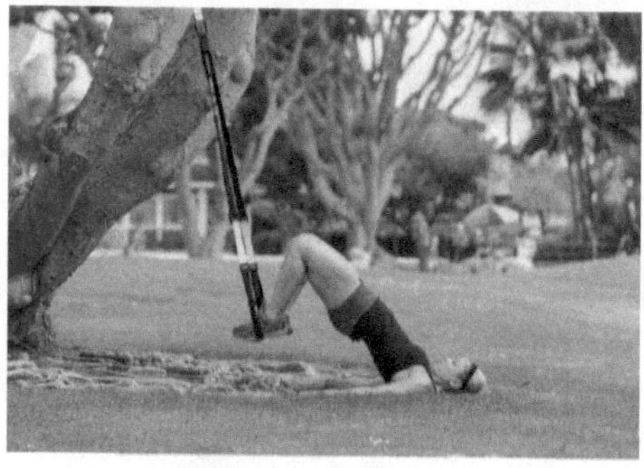

Hip Hinge

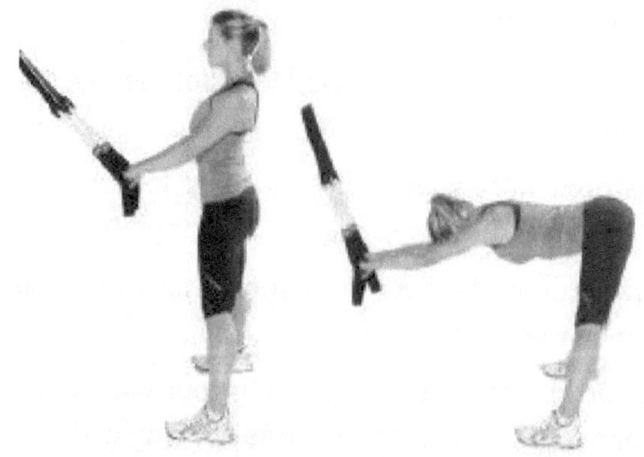

TRX Body Saw

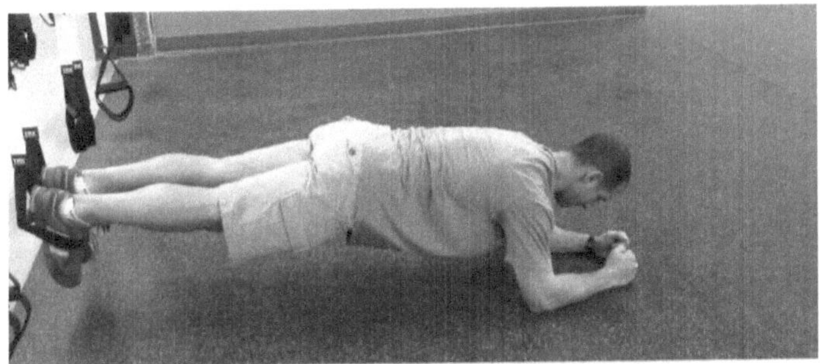

Setup: Adjust the TRX so the lowest point of the foot cradles is 8 to 12 inches from the ground.

Start position: Place your toes in floor.

TRX Pike

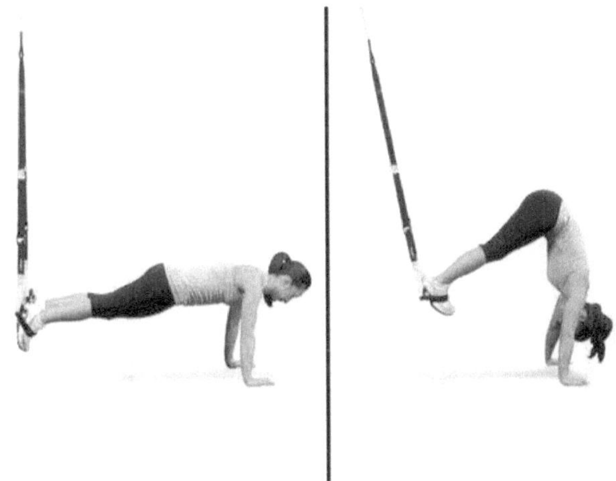

Setup: Adjust the TRX so the lowest point of the foot cradles is 8 to 12 inches from the ground.

Start here: Place your toes in floor.

TRX Rotating Hip and Back Stretch

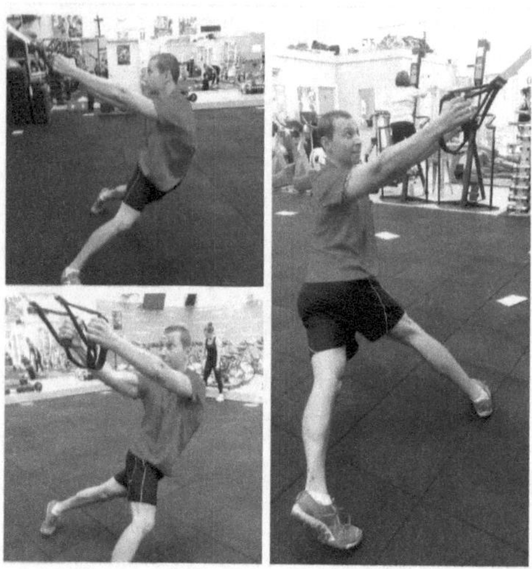

TRX Side Plank

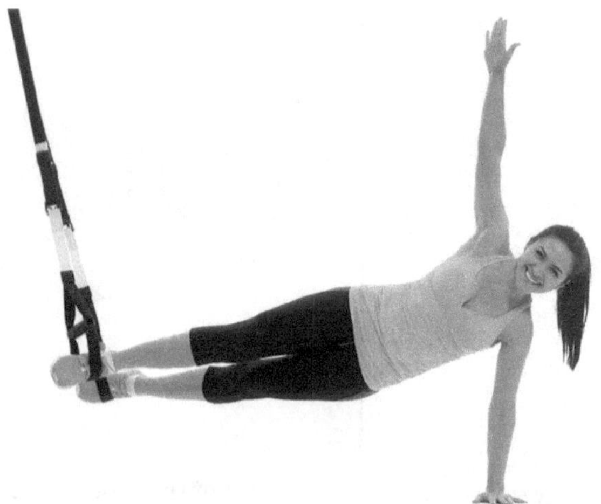

TRX Leg Bent Raises

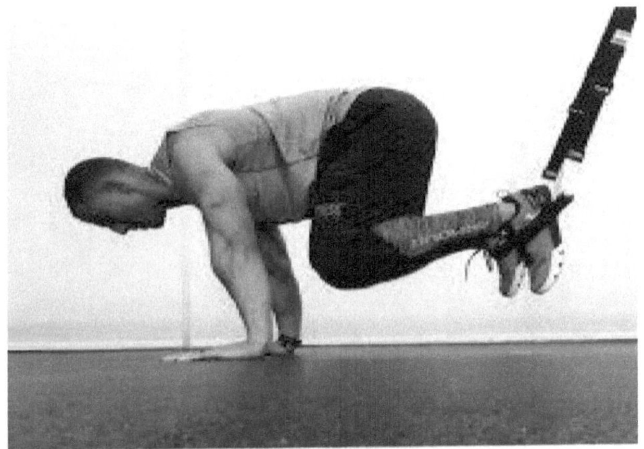